Principles
of
Biliary Lithotripsy

—edited by—

Alexander S. Cass, M.B.B.S.

Medical Director
Midwest Stone Management
Minneapolis, Minnesota;
Chief of Urology
Hennepin County Medical Center
Minneapolis, Minnesota

—and—

LeRoy H. Stahlgren, M.D., F.A.C.S.

Chief, General Surgery
St. Joseph's Hospital
Denver, Colorado;
Professor of Surgery
University of Colorado
Denver, Colorado

Judith Gunn Bronson, M.S.
Technical Editor

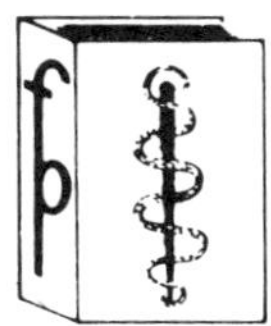

Futura Publishing Company, Inc.
Mount Kisco, New York
1989

Library of Congress Cataloging-in-Publication Data
Principles of biliary lithotripsy/edited by Alexander S. Cass and
    LeRoy H. Stahlgren.
        p. cm.
    Includes bibliographies and index.
    ISBN 0-87993-349-6
    1. Gallstones—Treatment. 2. Shock wave lithotripsy.   I.
Cass, Alexander.   II. Stahlgren, LeRoy H., 1924-
    [DNLM: 1. Biliary Tract Diseases—therapy.   2. Choleli-
thiasis—therapy.   3. Lithotripsy.   WI 750 P957]
RD547.P75   1989
617′ .556059—dc 19
DNLM/DLC
for Library of Congress   80-1108
                                             CIP

Copyright 1989
Futura Publishing Company, Inc.

Published by
Futura Publishing Company, Inc.
Bedford Ridge Road
Mount Kisco, New York 10507

L.C. no.: 89-1108
ISBN no.: 0-87993-349-6

Contributors

Henry C. Alder
Director
Division of Clinical Services and Technology
American Hospital Association
Chicago, Illinois

Craig H. Carpenter, M.D.
Director of Ultrasound
St. Joseph's Hospital
Denver, Colorado

Alexander S. Cass, M.B.B.S.
Medical Director
Midwest Stone Management
Minneapolis, Minnesota;
Chief of Urology
Hennepin County Medical Center
Minneapolis, Minnesota

Daniel H. Dunn, M.D.
General Surgeon
Abbott Northwestern Hospital
Minneapolis, Minnesota;
Clinical Assistant Professor of Surgery
University of Minnesota
Minneapolis, Minnesota

J. Kent Hamilton, M.D.
Department of Surgery
Section of Gastroenterology
Baylor University Medical Center
Dallas, Texas

Ronald C. Jones, M.D.
Chief
Department of Surgery
Baylor University Medical Center
Dallas, Texas

Paul Lubock, M.S.M.E.
Director of Engineering
Medstone International, Inc.
Costa Mosa, California

Robert D. Mackie, M.D.
Director
Biliary Center at
Abbott Northwestern Hospital
Minneapolis, Minnesota

J. Patrick O'Leary, M.D.
Seegar Chair in Surgery
Baylor University Medical Center
Dallas, Texas

LeRoy H. Stahlgren, M.D., F.A.C.S.
Chief, General Surgery
St. Joseph's Hospital
Denver, Colorado;
Professor of Surgery
University of Colorado
Denver, Colorado

David Vanderpool, M.D.
Attending Staff in Department of Surgery
Baylor University Medical Center
Dallas, Texas

Introduction

Health care professionals and patients alike are faced with an enormous task in keeping current with the profusion of new technologies that advance medicine's ability to manage problems. Biliary lithotripsy is such an advance.

Extracorporeal shock wave lithotripsy (ESL) was first used clinically for the treatment of renal stones in Munich, Germany, in 1980. A skeptical program committee of the American Urological Association rejected the Munich group's initial abstract for presentation at the Annual Meeting of the Association in 1982. However, by 1984, a Food and Drug Administration-approved trial of ESL for renal stones began at six centers in the United States, and ESL has since become the accepted treatment for most patients with renal and upper ureteral stones.

Biliary lithotripsy was also introduced in Munich, Germany (in 1985) and was approved by the FDA for trial in the United States beginning in January 1988. The editors have designed this text to satisfy the need for information early in biliary ESL's development phase. Topics of clinical relevance are addressed by authors who are themselves involved in planning, engineering, or clinical trials, with multiple investigational sites being represented. The basic, current information in these pages may lighten the burden on those desiring an overview of the fundamentals and a progress report of an evolving therapeutic modality.

Alexander S. Cass, M.B.B.S.
LeRoy H. Stahlgren, M.D.

Contents

1

The Physics and Mechanics of Lithotriptors

Paul Lubock

Introduction

The extracorporeal generation of shock waves for the noninvasive destruction of urinary tract stones was introduced clinically in the early 1980s. More recently, shock wave therapy has been extended for use in the biliary system. The first successful gallstone lithotripsy procedure in the United States under a Food and Drug Administration-approved protocol was performed in January 1988 using a Medstone 1050 ST system. Shock waves in this system are produced and focused by discharging a spark-gap electrode in a fluid-filled semi-ellipsoidal reflector.

Shock Wave Definition

The physical aspects governing the generation and propagation of shock waves can best be exemplified by examining the discharge of the spark-gap electrode as depicted in Figure 1. This discharge is effected by switching the electrical energy stored in a capacitor across the electrode

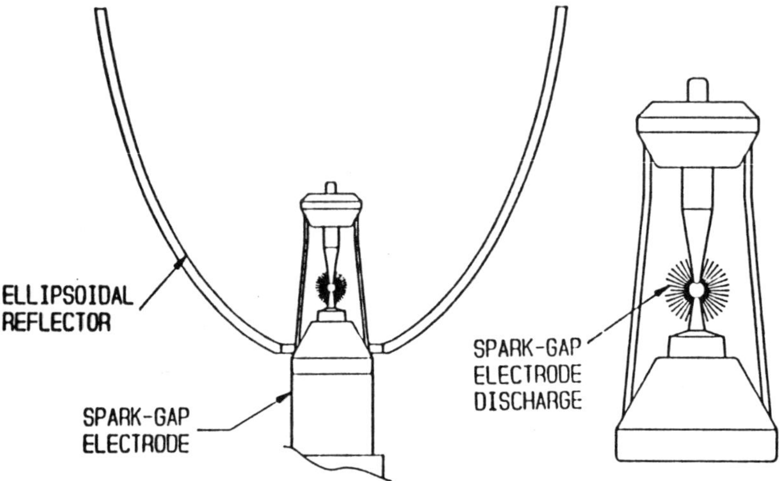

Figure 1: *Spark-gap electrode discharge in ellipsoidal reflector.*

tips, causing the rapid vaporization of fluid intimate to those tips. The resulting gaseous products expand violently in a radial fashion, forming a spherically symmetrical pressure disturbance, as shown in Figure 2.

Initially, the velocity at which this disturbance expands exceeds the velocity of sound in the fluid. The velocity of sound in a medium is the characteristic velocity at which small changes in pressure are transmitted from one point in the medium to another point. Table 1 lists the sound velocities of a number of fluids and materials.[1-4] Because the velocity of the expanding region is much greater than the velocity of sound in the fluid, its motion will not be detected immediately by the part of the fluid peripheral to the disturbed region. Therefore, a spherically expanding wave of compressed fluid will form at a higher density, pressure, and temperature than the fluid outside the diameter. This disturbed region is referred to as a shock front and propagates as a shock wave.

An idealized pressure versus time curve of a shock wave is shown in Figure 3A and is characterized by a steep rise time, typically on the order of tens of nanoseconds, followed

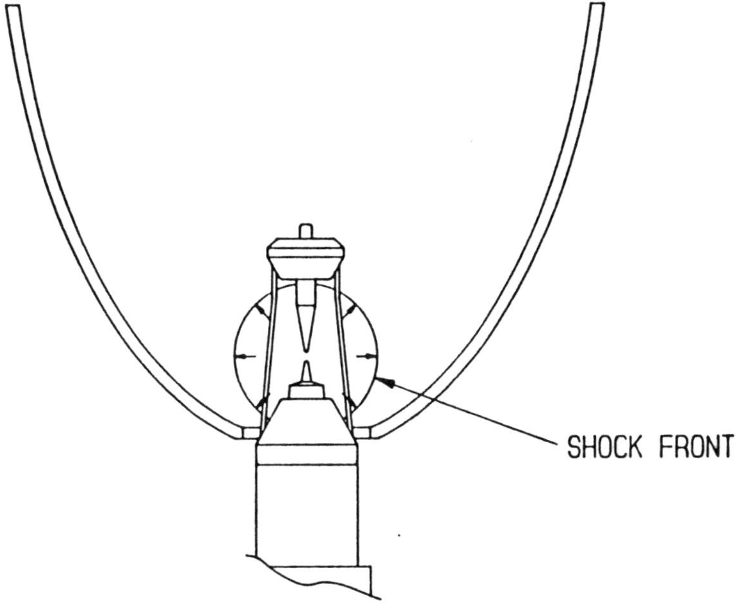

Figure 2: *Spherically symmetrical shock wave front.*

Table 1

Sound Velocities of Various Materials*

Materials	Sound Velocity (m/sec)
Air	330
Water	1500
Muscle	1545–1630
Fat	1460–1470
Kidney	1560
Urinary stone	6260
Gallstones	1400–2300
Brass	4400
Nickel	5600

*Data from references 1–4.

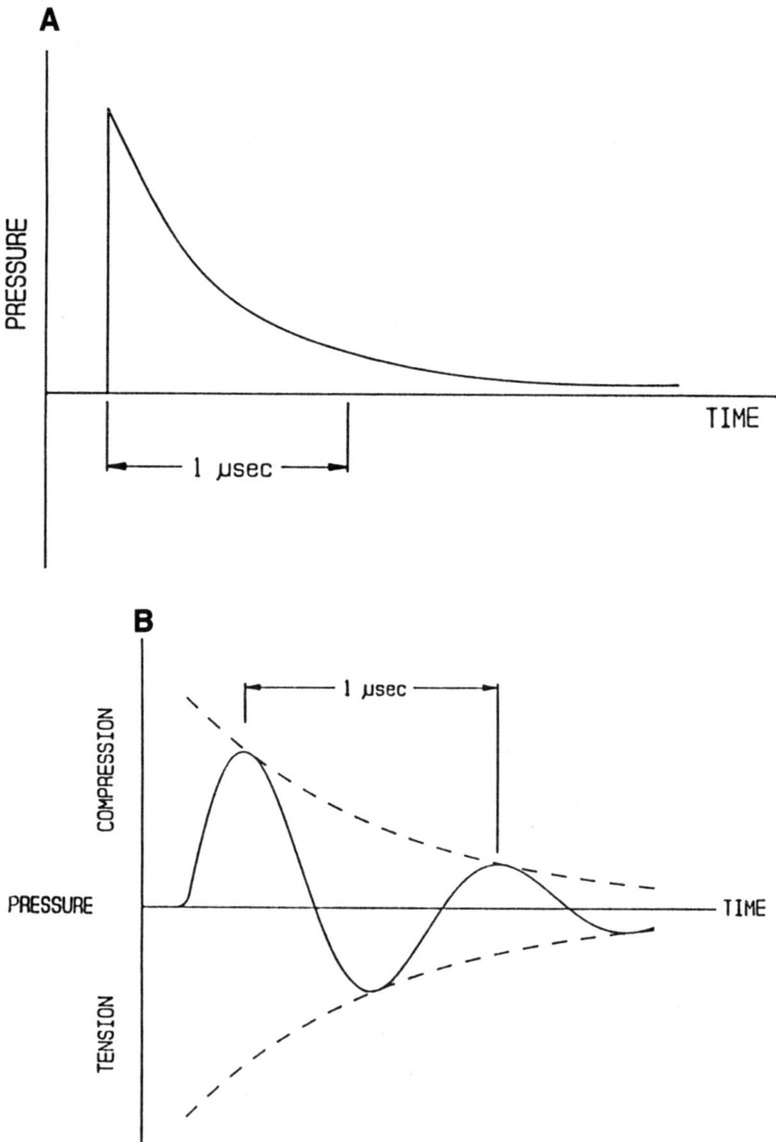

Figure 3: *Plots of pressure versus time. A. Shock wave. B. Ultrasound pulse.*

by an exponential decrease in pressure. This curve is easily distinguished from that of a typical ultrasound pulse, as shown in Figure 3B, which is sinusoidal, propagating at discrete frequencies with both positive (compressive) and negative (tensile) components of pressure. The negative components in the ultrasound pressure pulse waveform can lead to the formation and subsequent collapse of bubbles in fluids in a phenomenon known as *cavitation*. Further contrasts are apparent upon examination of the frequency spectrum of shock waves that contain different frequency components, many much lower than ultrasound frequencies.[5] This is significant because lower-frequency waves are able to pass through fluid and body tissues with minimal attenuation or damping. Therefore, shock waves are superior to ultrasound in penetrating tissues and delivering adequate pressures for stone destruction.

Shock Wave Reflection

When a shock wave strikes a dissimilar material, part of the wave is transmitted and part is reflected. For head-on or normal incidence, the proportions are given by:

$$P_t = [2Z_2/(Z_2 + Z_1)]Pi \qquad (1)$$
$$P_r = [(Z_2 - Z_1)/(Z_2 + Z_1)]Pi \qquad (2)$$
$$Z = \rho c \qquad (3)$$

where P_t is the transmitted pressure, Z is the acoustic impedance, P_i is the incident pressure, P_r is the reflected pressure, subscript 1 ($_1$) refers to the first material, subscript 2 ($_2$) refers to the second material, c is the velocity of sound in the material, and ρ is the density of the material.[6] A representation of this system is shown in Figure 4. Table 2 lists the densities and acoustic impedances of a number of materials and fluids.
Let us examine the head-on incidence of a plane 600-bar shock wave traveling in water ($Z_1 = 1.5$) as it collides with an idealized gallstone slab with an assumed acoustic impedance of 2.0 (Z_2), as schematically depicted in Figure 5. The transmitted pressure to the stone is approximately 686 bar, and the reflected pressure back to the water is approximately

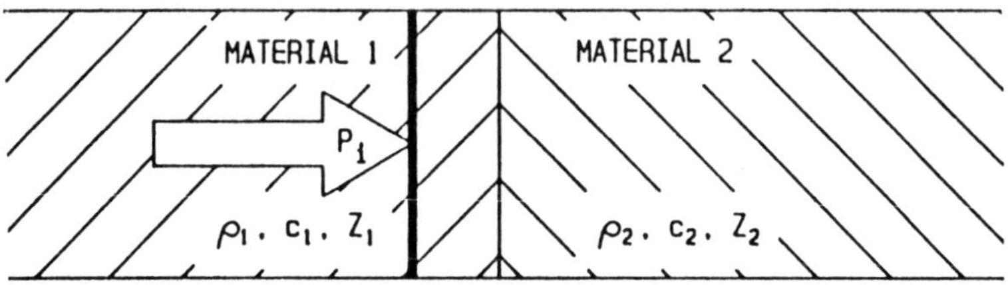

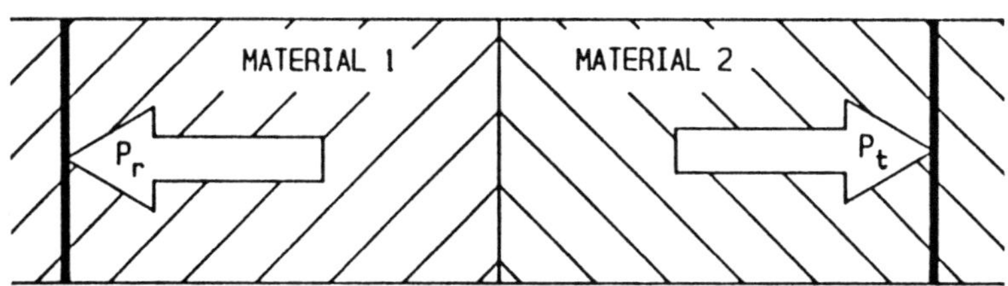

Figure 4: *Reflection of shock wave between dissimilar materials.*

Table 2

Densities and Acoustic Impedances of Various Materials*

Material	Density $10^3 \times kg/m^3$	Acoustic Impedance $10^6 \times kg/(m^2\ sec)$
Air	0.0012	0.0004
Water	1.0	1.5
Muscle	1.07	1.7
Fat	0.92	1.35
Kidney	1.04	1.62
Urinary stone	1.87	11.7
Gallstones	0.82–1.10	1.15–2.42
Brass	8.5	37.0
Nickel	8.9	49.5

*Data from references 1–4.

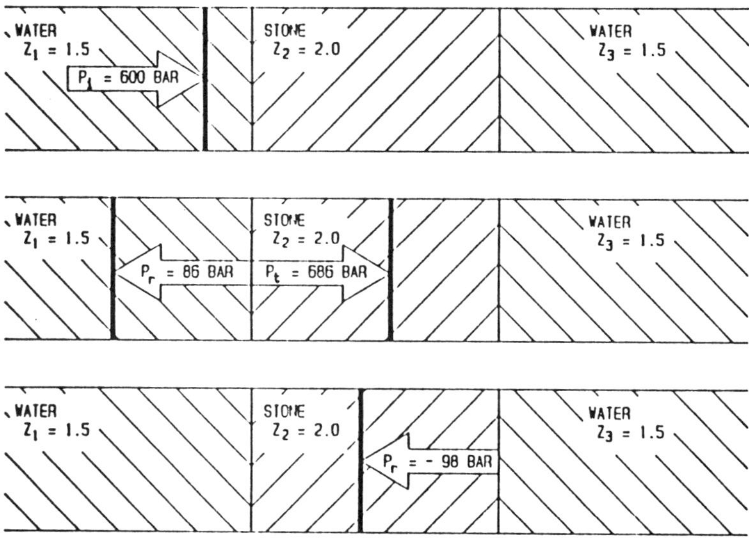

Figure 5: *Wave reflections on idealized gallstone slab.*

86 bar. Incident compressive shock waves may exceed the compressive strength of the stone; however, taking this example one step further, it can be shown that the 686-bar (compressive) pressure wave in the stone will reflect off the back surface of the stone as a tensile pressure wave of 98 bar. Because the compressive strengths of typical kidney stones and gallstones greatly exceed their tensile strengths, it is generally proposed that fractures of calculi from shock wave therapy are attributable to repeated tensile wave reflection. This fracture by the reflection of a high-intensity pressure wave is also known as *spalling*.

Other fracture mechanisms suggest that cavitation may play a role. For example, the reflected tensile wave in a calculus may reduce local pressures below the vapor pressure of the fluid (i.e., water) trapped or bonded within the calculus, causing the expansion of the fluid into a cavitation bubble. This rapid expansion or, more likely, the subsequent collapse of these bubbles might create stresses exceeding the fracture strength of the stone. Most theories suggest that the majority of cavitation damage is secondary to impacts from shock waves that radiate from the collapsing center of a bubble to an adjacent boundary or to the high stress caused by microjets of liquid impinging on adjacent boundaries during bubble collapse. Shear forces as well as cavitation induced around the stone have also been proposed as contributing mechanisms for stone fragmentation.

The reflection of a shock wave as it encounters an air interface is of particular concern because large negative pressures result secondary to the small acoustic impedance of air (i.e., $Z_2 = 0.0004$). For this reason, special precautions are taken to prevent tissue damage by avoiding shock wave encounter with tissue/gas interfaces such as those found in the lung and intestines as well as the shock wave entrance and exit areas.

Shock Wave Focusing

When there is oblique incidence of curved fronted shock waves onto nonplanar surfaces, the problem of shock wave reflection becomes more complex, as shear waves are also introduced and nonlinear reflections can occur.[6] However, classic geometry is adequate in describing the first order behavior of shock waves in lithotriptors. In fact, as previously mentioned, fluid-filled semi-ellipsoidal shells have proved to be an effective means of reflecting and focusing spherically fronted shock waves emanating from a spark-gap electrode discharged at the focal point. Shock waves striking the shell surface reflect and converge on and around the second geometric phantom focal point, referred to as F_2, whereas the initial spherical wave is blocked by the electrode endcap in the Medstone design to prevent unfocused energy from entering the patient, as shown in Figure 6. The pressure wave convergence results in the highest pressures being found in the vicinity of F_2. Increasing the aperture diameter of the shell increased the convergence angle at which focusing occurs and results in a decrease in pressure density as the waves exit. This technique is used to reduce the pressure level as waves pass through body tissues in an attempt to reduce patient pain perception.

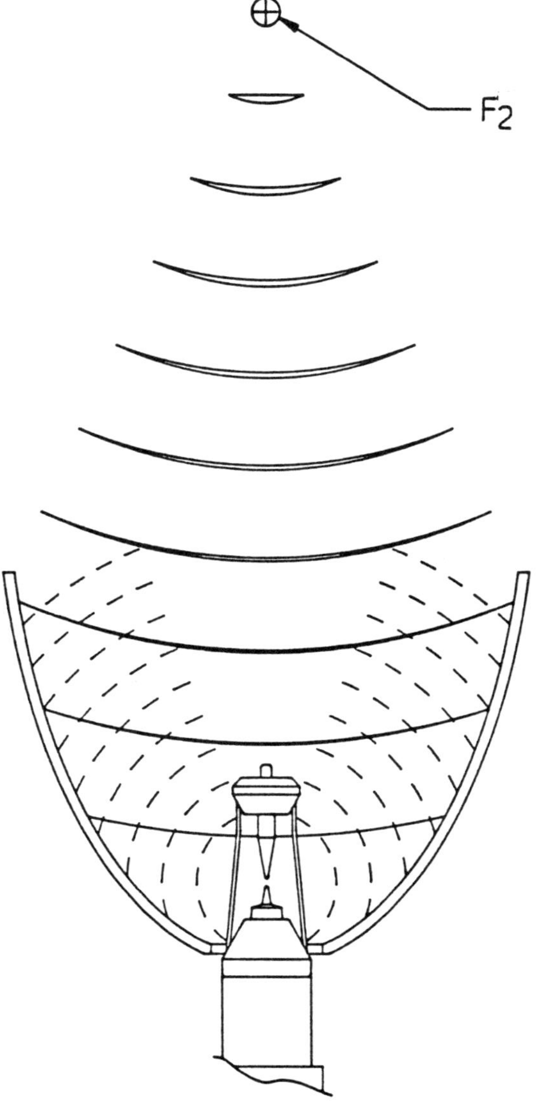

Figure 6: *Reflector focuses shock waves to second focal point (F₂).*

Shock Wave Pressure Measurement

The most common method of measuring relative shock wave pressures involves the use of piezoelectric transducers. These transducers contain materials such as tourmaline, quartz, or polyvinylidene fluoride because of their ability to produce an electrical potential in proportion to the amount of applied mechanical strain. Thus, when a shock wave passes through a piezoelectric transducer, a resulting voltage can be recorded. The absolute value of the shock wave pressure in lithotriptors cannot be determined with certainty, however, because of the following limitations:

1. interference by acoustic reflections from shock waves entering and exiting the transducer element;

2. the inability of transducer manufacturers to calibrate the transducer in a comparable underwater environment;

3. the lack of validated experimental evidence defining the charge sensitivity and acoustic constants of the transducer material under lithotriptor conditions;

4. interference with the propagation of the shock wave by the transducer package;

5. limited bandwidth of the charge-sensitive amplifiers processing the transducer signal;

6. strong dependence of the pressure on the alignment of the transducer surfaces to the shock front;

7. shock-induced spurious responses secondary to oblique incidence, shock diffraction, and edge effects; and

8. partial spalling damage to the transducer with subsequent loss of long-term stability after repeated shock exposure.[7]

There are also other application difficulties because of the unique measurement environment presented by the lithotriptor, and because of these problems, no standardized method has been universally accepted. Nevertheless, the pressure in the fluid at F_2 has been estimated to be between 300 and 900 bars. These pressures are effective for stone destruction.

Relative shock wave pressures were measured on the Medstone 1050 ST system using a tourmaline pressure transducer whose position was varied in the F_2 region. A

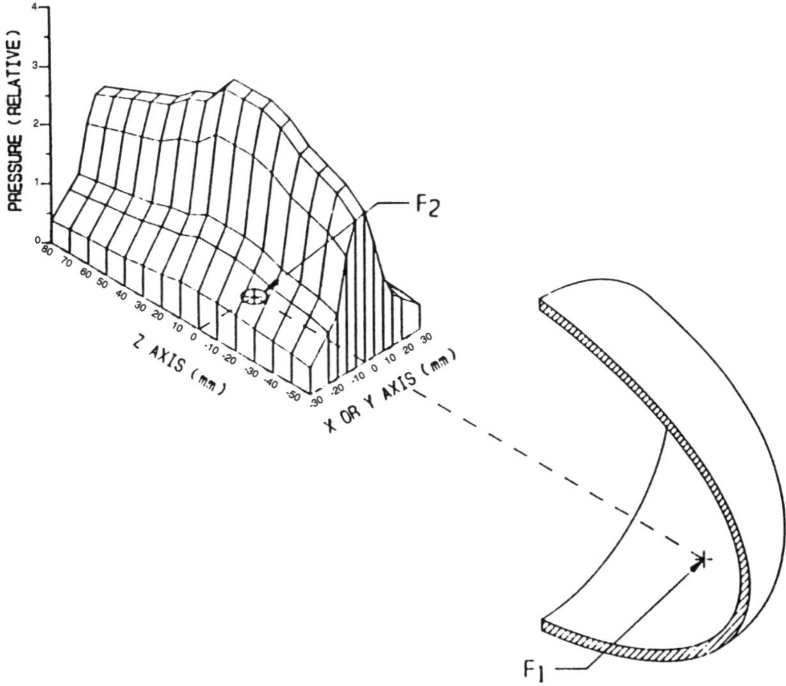

Figure 7: *Relative-pressure mapping at F_2.*

mapping of the results, as shown in Figure 7, indicates that the higher pressures are located along the Z-axis, near geometric F_2, with peak pressures skewed slightly toward the shock wave generation point (F_1). Pressure decreases more rapidly along the X and Y axes than along the Z axis.

Alternative Methods of Shock Wave Generation

Methods other than the spark-gap electrode generator system are being developed and used. These include microexplosive, laser, piezoelectric, and electromagnetic devices.

The microexplosive device generates shock waves by successive ignition of lead azide pellets in an ellipsoidal reflector.[8,9] There is a higher retreatment rate with this device that is probably attributable to lower pressures and longer pressure pulse width durations as well as to inconsistent firing. Special handling, storage, and disposal problem are involved with the explosive pellets.

Devices in which shock waves are produced by impulsively firing laser beams at F_1 in ellipsoidal reflectors have also been explored but are no longer being pursued for a number of reasons.[10] The problems include reliability, the cost of the laser source and components, and difficulties passing beams through fluid unimpeded by particulates and cavitation bubbles.

Piezoelectric devices produce shock waves by electrically pulsing hemispherical mosaics of piezoelectric material.[11,12] The subsequent rapid displacement of the piezoelectric elements causes pressure waves to converge at the hemisphere center. The energy levels attained by these devices are again much lower than those found in the spark-gap devices, and therefore retreatment rates have been higher, as have the number of shocks required for adequate fragmentation.

Electromagnetic devices are based on the principle that a force is exerted on a conductor carrying current in a magnetic field. Current-induced forces can therefore be directed to initiate pressure pulses in fluid, which are focused using acoustic lenses.[13,14] As with the piezoelectric devices, the number of shocks required to obtain adequate fragmentation has been much higher with this device than with spark-gap generators, as has the retreatment rate. Again, this is probably attributable to lower energy levels and extended pulse durations.

Shock Wave Coupling

The first lithotriptors coupled shock waves to the patient by immersing the patient while sitting, semisupine, in a large water bath.[15] This arrangement has obvious problems such as patient handling, general and emergency access difficulties, anesthetic delivery and ventilation difficulties, adverse effects on the cardiovascular system, monitoring problems, and the large space requirements for the bath, water processing plant, and patient-handling equipment.

The first human treatment with a "dry" shock wave lithotriptor occurred in October 1985 using a Medstone system. In this system, a fluid-filled flexible bellows was used to couple the shock wave generator to a plastic porthole in a flat radiographic table. The patient was coupled to the porthole using a water bag and mineral oil. Later, the water bag was found to be necessary only for thin patients, and most treatments are now performed using a film of mineral oil applied between the patient's skin and the porthole. A schematic of the coupling system is shown in Figure 8.

The design of the Medstone coupling system allows the shock wave to pass virtually unimpeded into the patient because of proper acoustic matching and selection of materials. These materials are also chosen and fabricated to

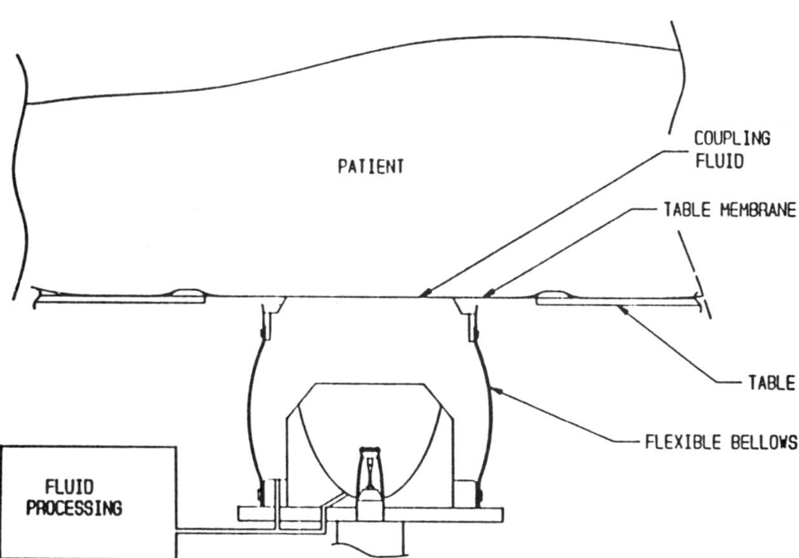

Figure 8: *Fluid coupling system with Medstone "dry" lithotriptor.*

withstand the harsh environment presented by repeated shock wave applications. The system controls conductivity, performs degassing, and removes gaseous by-products of the spark-gap discharge from the shock wave path to prevent energy absorption.

Other coupling systems include smaller water baths and pressurized bags isolated to the shock wave entrance area.

Stone Imaging and Localization

Three types of imaging techniques are employed for localizing stones: x-ray film, fluoroscopy, and ultrasound. For urinary tract stones, x-ray film provides the best-quality images. Fluoroscopic images can be difficult to obtain, particularly with large patients and low-density stones. As a result, exposure times are prolonged, increasing radiation exposure to the patient and personnel in the treatment room. Ultrasound imaging of kidney stones and fragments smaller than 4 mm as well as of ureteral stones is extremely difficult; however, for noncalcified biliary stones, ultrasound imaging is the modality of choice.

The Medstone 1050 ST provides x-ray film imaging for urinary tract stones and ultrasound imaging for biliary stones and radiolucent kidney stones. A schematic of the system is shown in Figure 9. The ultrasound system employs a hand-held freely moving ultrasound probe that is used to locate the biliary stone in conjunction with an overhead video system. The computer performs digital imaging analysis and uses a triangulation scheme to provide the operator with information allowing him to position the stone at F_2. This system allows real-time monitoring of the stone during fragmentation.

The x-ray system consists of an overhead tube, Bucky tray, and oblique film cassettes. The Bucky tray is used to take initial scout anteroposterior films for gross stone location. Oblique films, one cephalad and a second caudad, are taken and digitized. As in the ultrasound system, the computer can then, through a triangulation scheme, provide the operator with information to position the stone at F_2.

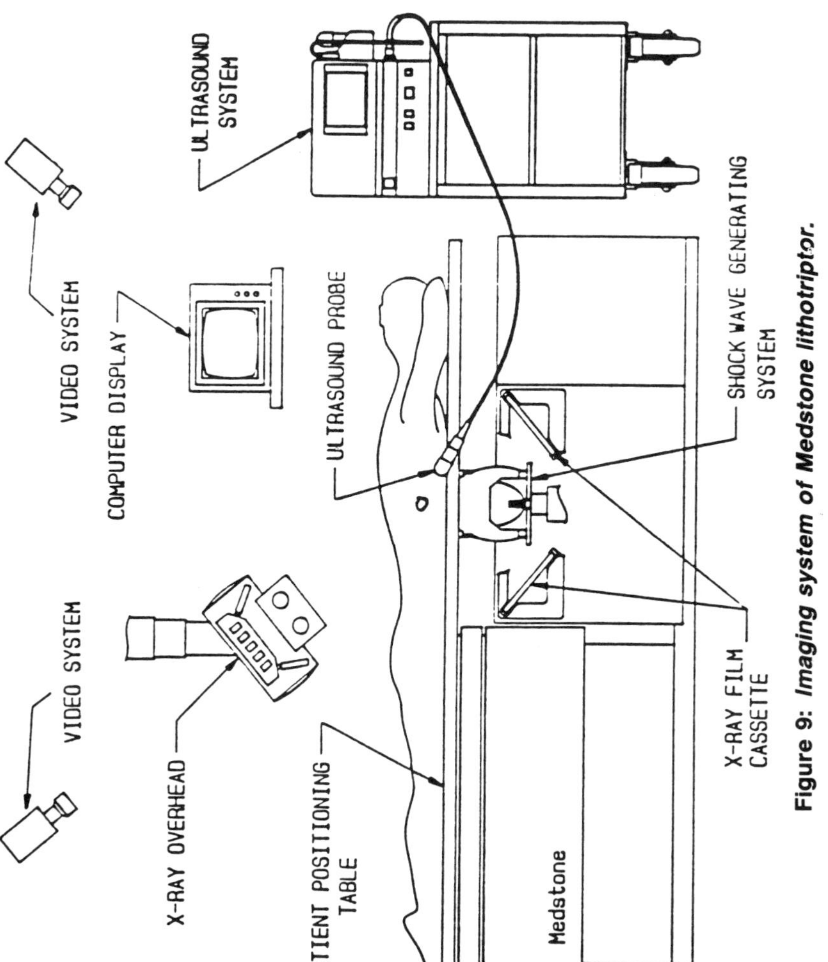

Figure 9: *Imaging system of Medstone lithotriptor.*

Fragmentation and treatment completion are determined by taking additional films.

Other systems use ultrasound probes attached to articulated arms capable of translational and rotational motion. These arms contain transducers from which the location of the stone is determined by computer. The summation of tolerances for each transducer must be accurately maintained for stone localization.

Conclusion

Future optimization of lithotriptor systems and subsystems will arise from a better understanding of the physical aspects of the shock wave and fragmentation process. This requires the determination of optimal pressure levels, densities, rise times, and decays to account for patient and stone variations. Technological improvements in localization modalities will also help increase overall effectiveness.

References

1. Wells PNT: *Biomedical Ultrasonics.* New York: Academic Press, 1977, p 124.
2. Katz JL: Elastic properties of urinary stones: Some experimental and theoretical observations. Proceedings of the National Academy of Sciences, National Research Conference on Urolithiasis, Washington, DC, 1972.
3. Ludwig GD, Struthers FW: Considerations Underlying the Use of Ultrasound to Detect Gallstones and Foreign Bodies in Tissue, Naval Medical Research Institute, Report No. 4, Bethesda, 1949.
4. Weast RC (ed): *Handbook of Chemistry and Physics,* 67th edition. Cleveland: The Chemical Rubber Company, 1986.
5. Chaussy C: *Extracorporeal Shock Wave Lithotripsy: New Aspects in the Treatment of Kidney Stone Disease.* Munich: S Karger, 1982, p 4.
6. Rinehart JS: *Stress Transients in Solids.* Santa Fe: HyperDynamicS, 1975, p 74.
7. Hunter PT, Finlayson B, Hirko RJ, et al: Measurement of shock wave pressures used for lithotripsy. *J Urol* 1986; 136:733.

8. Kuwahara M, Kanbe K, Kurosu S, et al: Extracorporeal stone disintegration using explosive pellets as an energy source of underwater shock waves. *J Urol* 1986; 135:814.

9. Kuwahara M, Kanbe K, Kurosu S, et al: Clinical application of extracorporeal shock wave lithotripsy using microexplosions. *J Urol* 1987; 137:837.

10. Mayo ME, Chapman WH, Ansell JS: Progress report on the lasertripter (abstract). *J Urol* 1986; 135:160A.

11. Rocco F, DeCobelli O, Caimi D, et al: Treatment of kidney stones with EDAP LT.01 and Wolf Piezolith 2200 piezoelectric lithotriptors (abstract). Fourth Symposium on Shock Wave Lithotripsy: State of the Art, Indianapolis, 1988.

12. Preminger GM: Piezoelectric lithotripsy: Wolf Piezolith 2200 (abstract). Fourth Symposium on Shock Wave Lithotripsy: State of the Art, Indianapolis, 1988.

13. Reichenberger WDM, Noske E, Riedmiller H, et al: New generation multifunctional shock wave lithotripter (abstract). *J Urol* 1986; 135:160A.

14. Jenkins AD: University of Virginia Lithostar experience (abstract). Fourth Symposium on Shock Wave Lithotripsy: State of the Art, Indianapolis, 1988.

15. Chaussy C: *Extracorporeal Shock Wave Lithotripsy: New Aspects in the Treatment of Kidney Stone Disease*. Munich: S Karger, 1982, p 96.

2

Present Use of Renal Lithotriptors

●

Alexander S. Cass

Introduction

The noninvasive procedure of lithotripsy fragments stones with shock waves, eliminating the need for traditional methods such as surgery. The technique was first used clinically in Germany in 1980 against kidney stones and was approved in the United States by the Food and Drug Administration (FDA) in December of 1984 after a 1-year United States clinical trial. To date, more than 1,000,000 patients worldwide have been treated with extracorporeal shock wave lithotripsy (ESL) for renal stones. Because experience with this first type of ESL is so extensive, it is worth reviewing as a means of gaining a perspective on the clinical utility and effects of ESL.

Equipment

The first-generation machine was the Dornier HM3 lithotriptor which requires a patient to be immersed in a tub of water through which the shock waves are transmitted (Fig. 1). The patient is usually given general, spinal, or epidural anesthetic, although local anesthesia injected subcutaneously at the skin entry site of the shock waves has

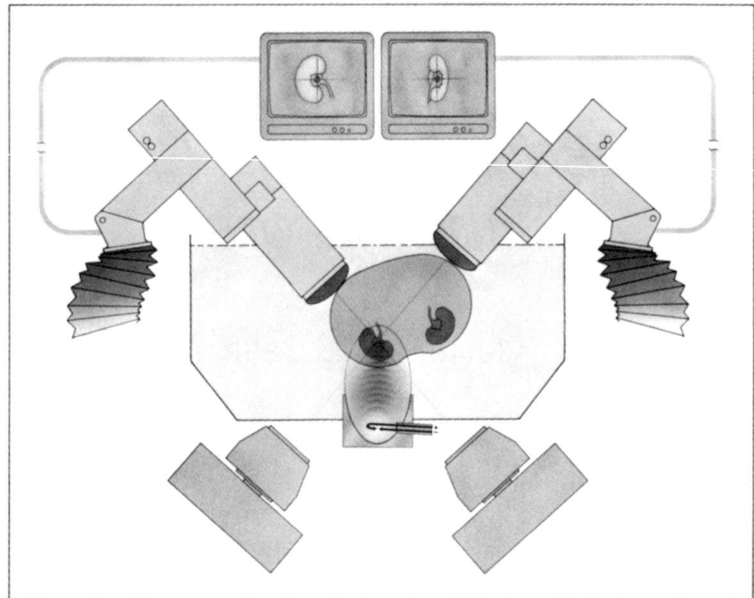

Figure 1: *First-generation lithotriptor (Dornier HM-3).*

been used in some centers. Initially, because of the high cost of the equipment, the patients often had to travel considerable distances to one of the larger centers that had purchased these units. However, in 1986, the FDA approved the mobile use of the Dornier HM3 lithotriptor and mobile renal lithotriptors began to operate. The advantage of such units is that the patient did not have to travel so far, since urologists in outlying areas can use the mobile unit on their patients in their own hometowns. There are concerns about quality control with the unit being operated by occasional users of lithotripsy instead of in a fixed site where the closed staff used the lithotriptor on a more regular basis. These concerns are addressed in the *Results* section of this chapter.

Medstone International developed the first of the second-generation machines, a tubless lithotriptor in the United States; and in 1985, its FDA-approved investigational trial started. In this machine, the patient is coupled to the shock wave generator by a fluid-filled bag and mineral oil between adjoining surfaces (Fig. 2). There is a re-

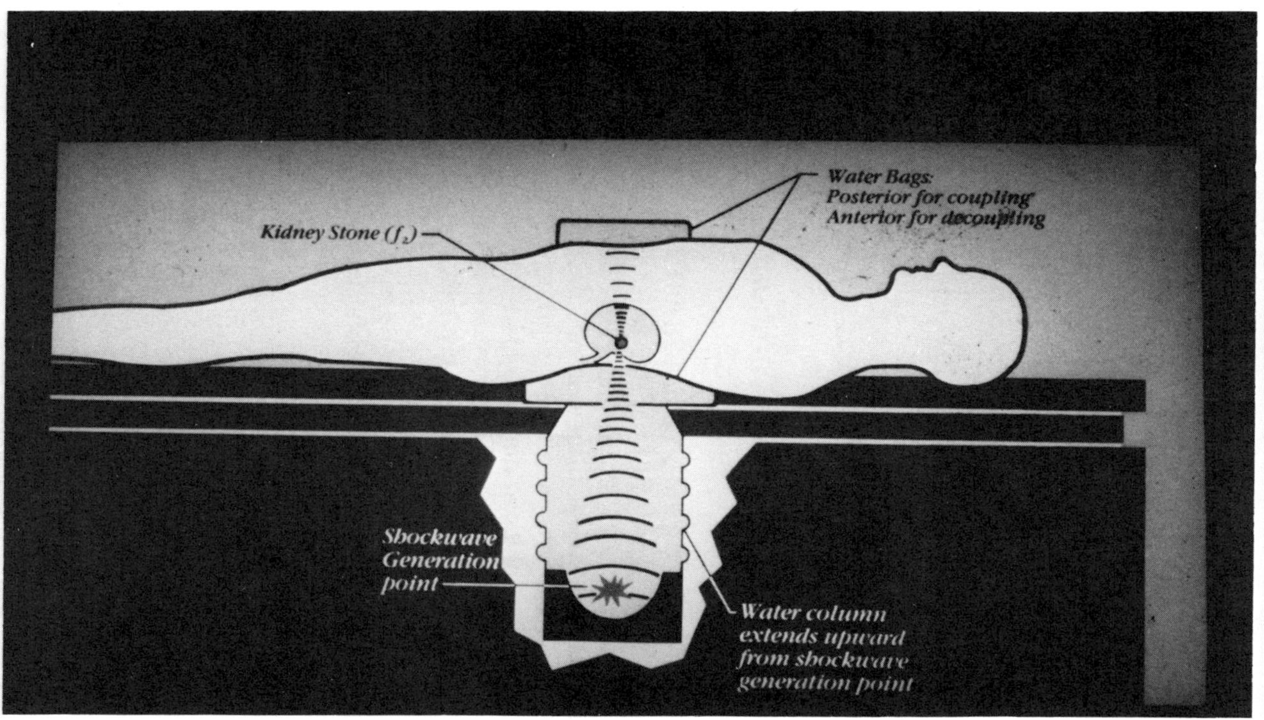

Figure 2: *Second-generation lithotriptor (Medstone).*

duced need for anesthesia with some second-generation lithotriptors, with many patients requiring none at all, because of the lower total energy force being generated by the lithotriptor. However, more shocks are required for disintegration of renal stones, and the rate of repeat treatments to achieve satisfactory fragmentation is much higher than when a higher total force energy is used. The source of the shock wave has also been changed, from the original spark-gap generation to electromagnetic force or piezoelectric generation. The method of localizing the stone is by x-ray imaging in the first-generation machine; some second-generation machines are using ultrasound (Table 1).

Which Patients are Candidates for Renal ESL?

Between 90% and 95% of patients with calculi located in the kidney and upper ureter are now eligible for ESL. Stones as large as 3 cm in diameter can be treated by ESL alone; patients with kidney stones greater than 3 cm will normally require a percutaneous procedure in combination with ESL although some urologists use repeat ESL alone. Patients with stones 1.5 to 3 cm in diameter can have a double-J ureteral stent passed prior to ESL that allows the passage of the many fragments without causing ureteral obstruction, thus obviating a secondary post-ESL procedure. Nonopaque stones can be treated by injecting contrast medium during the procedure via a previously passed ureteral catheter, which will allow monitoring of the stone and its fragments during the procedure. Ureteral stones are manipulated into the kidney prior to lithotripsy.

The procedure may not be practical in cases where there is an obstructive abnormality in the urinary tract distal to the stone. Extracorporeal lithotripsy is contraindicated in pregnant patients and patients with bleeding disorders. Patients weighing more than 300 pounds are not candidates with the first-generation lithotriptor but are suitable for the second-generation machines.

Table 1
Characteristic Features of Various Lithotriptors

Manufacturer	Generation	Focusing	Coupling	Localization	Positioning
Dornier HM3	Spark gap	Ellipsoid	Bath	Biplane fluoro	Move patient
Dornier HM4	Spark gap	Ellipsoid	Membrane	Biplane fluoro	Move patient
EDAP LT-01	Piezoelectric	Spherical	Membrane	Ultrasound	Move generator
Medstone 1050	Spark gap	Ellipsoid	Membrane	Plain films	Move patient
Northgate	Spark gap	Ellipsoid	Membrane	Ultrasound	Move reflector
Siemens Lithostar	Two electro-magnetic	Acoustic lens	Membrane	Two fluoroscopes	Move generator
Technomed Sonolith 3000	Spark gap	Ellipsoid	Pool	Ultrasound	Move generator
Wolf Piezolith 2200	Piezoelectric	Spherical	Pool	Ultrasound	Move patient
Yashiyoda	Microexplosive	Ellipsoid	Bath	C-scan x-ray	Move x-ray

Post-ESL Treatment

In most patients, the majority of the stone particles produced by ESL pass out of the body during the first 2 to 4 weeks after treatment. Renal colic of various degrees will necessitate the use of narcotic analgesia in about one-third of patients for the first few days, and a small percentage of these patients will require admission to the hospital. All patients will pass blood in the urine for several days after lithotripsy.

Outpatient follow-up of the asymptomatic patient consists of an examination on post-treatment day 21 with an abdominal plain radiograph (KUB), blood pressure measurement, and urinalysis. If the patient is stone-free and infection-free at this visit, he or she is discharged. If the patient is asymptomatic and the radiograph shows some fragments remaining, the patient returns at 3 months for the same investigations. If the patient is symptomatic, for example, in pain, or if the radiograph shows a moderate to a large number of fragments remaining, or if urinary infection is present, examination takes place at 14-day intervals until the majority of fragments have passed and the patient is free of infection. This follow-up regimen will diagnose the post-ESL complication of a nonfunctioning kidney due to persistent asymptomatic obstruction or obstructed pyelonephritis with urosepsis, which require secondary procedures.

Results and Complications of ESL

Initial Results with Fixed-Site Machines

Two large series of patients treated in fixed-site Dornier HM3 lithotriptor units in the United States have been published. The first is the 1985 report of the American Urological Association's Ad Hoc Committee, which encompasses almost 4,000 patients treated at six institutions. Of these patients, 88% had required a single ESL session, 13% had required a post-ESL procedure, and 76% to 95% were stone-free at 2 to 3 months (Table 2).[1] Because these were the

Table 2
Comparison of Results of Fixed and Mobile Unit Lithotriptors

No. Pts.	No. ESL Sessions (%)			Procedures Post-ESL (%)	Av. Postop. Stay (Days)	No or Insignificant Stones at F/U (%)
	1	2	3			
3943*†	81	11	1	13	4	76–95
1030*‡	90	9	1	10	2.8	96
1120**	92	7	1	5.5	1.1	92

* Fixed lithotriptor.
† Data from reference 1.
‡ Data from reference 2.
** Author's data with mobile unit.

first cases performed in the United States, subsequent results can be expected to be better. Indeed, Lingeman and associates treated 1,030 renal units, with 90% of patients requiring a single ESL session, 10% requiring a post-ESL procedure, and most patients either being stone-free at follow-up (72%) or having only clinically insignificant fragments (24%) (Table 2).[2]

Results with Mobile Machines

Our results with a mobile lithotriptor used at multiple sites by many properly trained urologists are similar. Our mobile Dornier HM3 lithotriptor started operation on September 24, 1986, and had performed 1,209 treatments on 1,002 patients by December 31, 1987. The stone location and size are summarized in Table 3. Almost all patients received general anesthesia. Ureteral stones were manipulated into the kidney with a double-J ureteral stent inserted via cystoscopy either a few days prior to ESL (155 patients, 15.5%) or at the time of ESL (64 patients, 6%). An indwelling double-J ureteral stent was passed via cystoscopy either prior to ESL (320 patients, 32%) or at the time of ESL (119 patients, 12%). In 160 patients (16%), a ureteral catheter was inserted at the time of ESL for instillation of contrast medium to aid in the localization of the stone.

The average time of ESL was 51 minutes for a single stone and 61 minutes for multiple stones. The average number of shocks was 1,598 for a single stone and 1,974 for multiple stones. The average radiation dose to the patient was 17 rads with a single stone and 23 rads with multiple stones. The ESL was performed as same-day surgery in 207 patients (22%) whereas 671 patients (71.5%) spent the night after ESL in the hospital. Only 61 (6.5%) required 2 days or more of hospitalization. The length of hospitalization was not recorded in the remaining 63 patients.

The ESL treatment was repeated once in 80 renal units (7%) and twice in nine renal units (1%). Secondary procedures for the removal of stone fragments were performed in 64 renal units (6%) and consisted of transurethral endoscopic ureteral manipulation in 28, indwelling double-J

Table 3
Stone Localization and Size in Relation to ESL Treatments Given

	Single Stone No. (%)	Multiple Stones No. (%)	TOTAL
LOCATION			
Pelvis	356 (51.3)	177 (30)	
Calix—Upper	51 (7.4)	94 (16)	
—Middle	28 (4)	74 (12.5)	
—Lower	176 (25.3)	197 (33.5)	
Ureter—Upper	80 (11.6)	39 (7)	
—Middle	2 (0.2)	0	
—Lower	2 (0.2)	5 (1)	
	695 pts	586 (307 pts)	
SIZE (CM)			
<1	348 (48)	122 (40)	
1–2	295 (40)	139 (45)	
2–3	67 (9)	31 (10)	
>3	19 (3)	15 (5)	
	729*	307	
TREATMENTS			
1	684 (94)	347 (89)	1031 (92)
2	39 (5)	41 (10)	80 (7)
≥3	6 (1)	3 (1)	9 (1)
	729 renal units	391 renal units	1120 renal units

*Bilateral single stones—34 patients

Table 3—Continued
Stone Localization and Size in Relation to ESL Treatments Given

	Single Stone No. (%)	Multiple Stones No. (%)	TOTAL
Average number of shocks	1598	1974	
Average radiation to patient (rads)	17	23	
Average time taken (minutes)	51	61	
HOSPITALIZATION			
Same day discharge	130 (19)	77 (25)	207 (22)
1 day	464 (67)	207 (67)	671 (71.5)
2 days	23 (3)	12 (4)	35 (4)
More than 2 days	15 (2)	11 (4)	26 (2.5)
Not known	63 (9)	—	—
	695 pts	307 pts	939 pts

ureteral stent passage via cystoscopy in 16, percutaneous nephrostomy or nephrolithotomy in 15, and open operation (ureterolithotomy or pyelolithotomy) in 5.

The 3-month films showed 552 of 741 renal units (74.5%) to be stone-free, 131 (17.5%) to have stone fragments less than 0.4 cm in diameter, and 58 (8%) to have asymptomatic fragments larger than 0.4 cm.

Special Strategies for Large Stones

With increasing experience, different strategies have evolved for the treatment of large stones (greater than 3 cm in diameter), such as partial or complete staghorn stones. Because of the large total stone burden, success with a single ESL treatment is the exception, in such cases.

Patients with large stone masses can be managed in a two-stage ESL procedure. At the initial treatment session, a double stent is inserted and left indwelling to prevent larger fragments of stone from falling into the ureter after the first ESL, which would necessitate a ureteral manipulation before the follow-up ESL session. A second session is then undertaken for destruction of the remaining stone mass. Fractionated disintegration in two or more ESL sessions is feasible in most cases of staghorn stones in a nondilated or mildly dilated collecting system without anatomic abnormalities. Because of the large stone burden, however, the period until the patient becomes stone-free is considerably prolonged.

As an alternative for staghorn stones with a very large stone mass in an enlarged collecting system, a percutaneous stone debulking procedure is performed. In a second session, usually after 2 to 4 days, ESL is employed to destroy the remaining caliceal stone parts. Ureteral manipulation of extended "Steinstrasse" (column of stone fragments in ureter) is being undertaken less frequently as the use of the double-J stent has greatly reduced the incidence.

Recurrence

Approximately 30% of patients having successful ESL still have small asymptomatic stone fragments within the kidney 3 months later. Although these fragments usually do not cause clinical complications such as obstruction, they may provide a nidus for more rapid regrowth of stone material. Current information indicates that the stone recurrence rate in patients who are rendered free of stones with ESL is 9% annually, whereas the rate is 22% in those patients with residual fragments.[3]

Clinical Side Effects of ESL

Although ESL is well tolerated by most patients, shock waves are not without observable biological effect. The most consistent alteration noted immediately following 200 shock waves is gross hematuria, which generally resolves within the first 12 hours.[4,5] Pain is also common and appears to be related to the number and size of the stones treated.[6] Additionally, significant rises in several serum and urinary values are seen 24 hours after ESL: bilirubin, lactic dehydrogenase, serum glutamic asparate transferase (SGOT), creatinine phosphokinase, N-acetyl-beta-glucosaminidase, beta-galactosidase, and gamma-glutamyl transpeptidase.[6-10] These data imply that there is significant trauma to the kidney and adjacent tissues (liver, skeletal muscle). Most of these laboratory values begin to fall within 3 to 7 days and are normal at 3 months.

Other organ systems have also been damaged during ESL. The lung parenchyma can be damaged if directly exposed to shock waves.[11] Several cases of clinically typical acute pancreatitis associated with a marked rise in serum amylase and lipase levels have been observed.[7] Also, an increase in amylase levels has been reported in the absence of manifest pancreatitis.[7] In addition, it is recognized that shock waves can induce extrasystoles, thus necessitating ECG synchronization with R-wave triggering on the Dornier HM3 device.

Renal Injury During ESL

Clinical Findings

The renal trauma produces effects ranging from mild contusions localized in the parenchyma to large hematomas associated with severe bleeding that may necessitate blood transfusion and arteriographic embolization.[5,12,13]

The two most common side effects seen shortly after ESL are hemorrhage and edema within or around the kidney. Perirenal and subcapsular fluid (blood or urine) accumulation has been reported in as many as 24% to 32% of patients. This fluid is reabsorbed within a few days to a few weeks after the lithotripsy.[5]

A recent study by Knapp and associates found that patients with existing hypertension are more likely to develop perinephric hematomas.[14] In particular, those patients having unsatisfactory control of their hypertension at the time of treatment had the highest incidence of hematomas. Those workers evaluated the number of shock waves, accelerating voltage, and "power" (number of shock waves $\times$ accelerating voltage) as potential risk factors and found no correlation with the onset of hematomas. It is interesting to speculate whether other underlying disease processes are also potential risk factors in ESL treatment.

Other renal changes commonly noted after ESL are enlargement and a loss of corticomedullary demarcation.[5,13-15]

Both of these changes suggest damage to either the nephron or the renal vasculature sufficient to cause extravasation of blood or urine into the extracellular space. Such edema could compress structures within the kidney, resulting in chronic interstitial and tubular scarring.

Experimental Studies

There have been only a few animal studies published that document the bioeffects of shock waves generated during ESL. These studies demonstrate structural and functional changes after shock wave administration that correlate well with the side effects observed in patients.

Studies performed in dogs have identified both acute and chronic changes.[16-19] The acute alterations appear primarily in the kidney and are similar to those that occur in patients. Kidney enlargement and hematuria are the most commonly detected changes. Interstitial edema may involve the entire kidney, whereas areas of hemorrhage appear to be more focal. Hemorrhage has been found in three general areas: perirenal, subcapsular, and intraparenchymal. Hematomas ranging in size from minute to 0.5 cm in diameter have been reported. Delius and co-workers performed a morphological analysis of renal injury in ESL-treated dogs and observed that the number and size of the hematomas were related to the number of shock waves administered to the kidney.[19] That is, greater change was induced by 1,500 to 3,000 shock waves than by 500 shock waves. Tissue injury included damage to the thin-walled veins.[18,19] Venous thrombi were also frequent in the interlobular and arcuate veins located at the sites of hemorrhage.[19] Most of these alterations were reversible in several weeks, except for some of the large hematomas. Delius and co-workers also found histological evidence of tubular injury localized to areas of intraparenchymal hemorrhage immediately after ESL.[19] Tubular changes consisted of dilation and cast formation and were generally restricted to the mid portion of the kidney, the renal poles being spared. However, in this study, shock waves had been focused on the renal pelvis, so the mid portion of the renal parenchyma was within the high-pressure field of the shock waves.

Only one study has followed the changes in serum enzyme levels and creatinine clearance after shock wave treatment. No alterations were noted for as long as 10 days following the administration of 500 shocks.[11] Focusing of shock waves on the intestine and liver produced petechial bleeding acutely but with no histological changes at 14 days.[11]

Chronic changes following shock wave treatment do not appear to be clearly known at this time. Newman and associates identified morphological changes in the dog kidney at 30 days after treatment.[18] These alterations consisted of diffuse interstitial fibrosis, focal areas of calcification, nephron loss, dilated veins, and hyalinized to acellular scars running from the cortex to the medulla. In contrast, Chaussy reported no histological abnormalities in dog kidneys up to 1 year after treatment.[11]

References

1. American Urological Association Ad Hoc Committee to Study the Safety and Clinical Efficacy of Current Technology of Percutaneous Lithotripsy and Noninvasive Lithotripsy: Report. Baltimore: American Urological Association, Inc, 1985.
2. Lingeman JE, Coury TA, Newman DM, et al: Comparison of results and morbidity of percutaneous nephrostolithotomy and extracorporeal shock wave lithotripsy. *J Urol* 1987; 138:485.
3. Newman DM, Scott JW: Long-term follow-up of 2,617 extracorporeal shock wave patients (abstract). *J Urol* 1987; 137:45A.
4. Chaussy C, Schmiedt E, Jocham D, et al: Extracorporeal shock wave lithotripsy (ESL) for treatment of urolithiasis. *Urology* 1984; 23:59.
5. Kaude JV, Williams MC, Millner MR, et al: Renal morphology and function immediately after extracorporeal shock wave lithotripsy. *AJR* 1985; 145:305.
6. Drach GW, Dretler S, Fair W, et al: Report of the United States Cooperative Study of Extracorporeal Shock Wave Lithotripsy. *J Urol* 1986; 135:1127.
7. Lingeman JE, Newman D, Mertz, JHO, et al: Extracorporeal shock wave lithotripsy: The Methodist Hospital of Indiana experience. *J Urol* 1986; 135:1134.
8. Ruiz-Marcellan FJ, Ibarz-Servio L: Evaluation of renal damage in extracorporeal lithotripsy by shock waves. *Eur Urol* 1986; 12:73.
9. Parr KL, Lingeman JE, Jordan M, Coury TA: Changes in creatinine kinase concentrations and electrocardiographic changes in extracorporeal shock wave lithotripsy. *Urology* 1988; 32:21.
10. Assimos DG, Boyce WH, Furr EG, et al: Urinary enzyme levels after extracorporeal shock wave lithotripsy (abstract). *J Urol* 1987; 137:45A.
11. Chaussy C: *Extracorporeal Shock Wave Lithotripsy: Technical Concepts, Experimental Research and Clinical Application.* Basel: S Karger, 1986.
12. Knapp PK, Scott J, Lingeman JE: Magnetic resonance imaging following extracorporeal shock wave lithotripsy with the Dornier HM3 lithotripter (abstract). *J Urol* 1987; 137:287A.
13. Rubin JI, Arger PH, Pollack HM, et al: Kidney changes after extracorporeal shock wave lithotripsy: CT evaluation. *Radiology* 1987; 162:21.
14. Knapp PM, Kulb TB, Lingeman JE, et al: Extracorporeal shock

wave lithotripsy induced perirenal hematomas. *J Urol* 1988; 139:700.

15. Grantham JR, Millner MR, Kaude JV, et al: Renal stone disease treated with extracorporeal shock wave lithotripsy: Short-term observations in 100 patients. *Radiology* 1986; 158:203.

16. Thibault P, Dory J, Cotard JP, et al: Lithotripsy by ultrashort pulsation: Experimental study in renal lithiasis in the dog. *Ann Urol (Paris)* 1986; 20:20.

17. Brendel W: Effect of shock waves on canine kidneys. In: Gravenstein JS, Peter K (eds): *Extracorporeal Shock Wave Lithotripsy for Renal Stone Disease: Technical and Clinical Aspects.* Stoneham: Butterworths, 1986, p 141.

18. Newman R, Hackett R, Senior D, et al: ESL: Pathologic effects on canine renal tissues. *Urology* 1987; 29:194.

19. Delius M, Enders G, Xuan Z, et al: Biological effects of shock waves: kidney damage by shock waves in dogs: Dose dependence. *Ultrasound Med Biol* 1988; 14:117.

3

The Biliary System and Stone Formation

●

Robert D. Mackie

Introduction

The biliary system for bile flow begins at the cellular level with small intercellular canaliculi. The remaining system encompasses the intrahepatic ducts, extrahepatic ducts, and gallbladder. The primary function of the system is to carry bile from the liver to the duodenum. Stone formation is the most common disorder, the mechanism of which is starting to be understood.

Physiology

Total daily bile flow in humans approximates 600 ml at a secretory pressure of approximately 23 mmHg. The principal components of the bile are water (82%), bile acids (12%), lecithin and other phospholipids (4%), and unesterfied cholesterol (0.7%). Lesser constituents include conjugated bilirubin, proteins (IgA and others), electrolytes, mucus, and, often, drugs and their metabolites.

Hepatic bile is a pigmented isotonic fluid with an electrolyte composition resembling that of blood plasma. In the gallbladder, most inorganic anions, including chloride and bicarbonate, have been removed by resorption across the basement membrane.

Three mechanisms are important in regulating bile flow: active transport of bile acids from hepatocytes into the canaliculi, bile acid–induced ATPase-mediated transport of sodium, and ductal secretion.

Bile acids are an important physiologic driving force for hepatic bile flow and aid in water and electrolyte transport in the small bowel. The primary bile acids, cholic and chenodeoxycholic acids, are synthesized from cholesterol in the liver, conjugated with glycine or taurine, and excreted into the bile. Secondary bile acids, including deoxycholate and lithocholate, are formed in the gut as bacterial metabolites of the primary bile acids. Other, tertiary, bile acids, including urosodeoxycholic acid (a stereoisomer of chenodeoxycholic acid), are found in only trace amounts in human bile.

Bile acids are detergents which, at normal ratios with lecithin and cholesterol, favor the formation of solubilizing mixed micelles. The concentrations may be expressed on triangular coordinates as in the classic phase diagram in Figure 1.[1] Abnormal ratios—above the equilibrium line—promote the precipitation of cholesterol crystals in the bile. In addition to facilitating the biliary excretion of cholesterol, bile acids are necessary for the normal intestinal absorption of dietary fats via a micellar transport mechanism.

Bile acids are efficiently conserved under normal conditions by two methods of reabsorption. First, they are passively absorbed along the entire gut. Second, and quantitatively much more important, is the active transport of conjugated bile acids in the distal ileum. The reabsorbed bile acids enter the portal bloodstream and are taken up avidly by the liver.

The normal bile acid pool contains approximately 2 to 4 g. After a meal, the bile acid pool undergoes one or more enterohepatic cycles, depending on the size and composition of the meal. Normally, the pool circulates approximately five to ten times daily. Although the loss of bile salts in the stool is usually matched by increased hepatic synthesis,

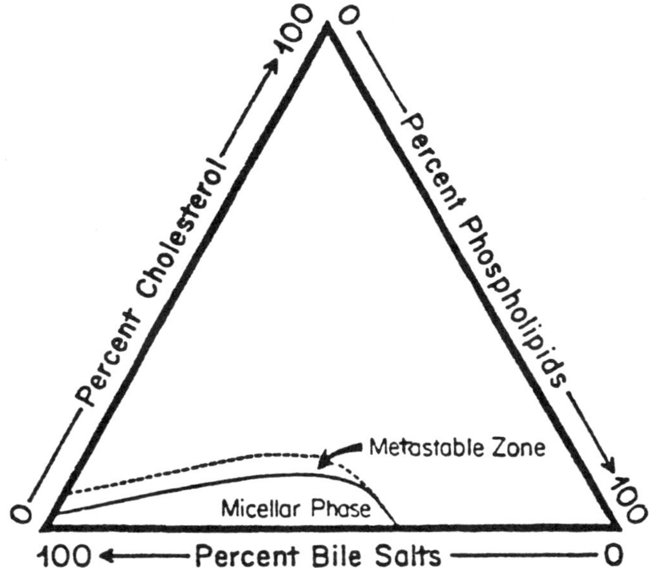

Figure 1: *Triangular coordinate plot of model bile. Shown are the metastable – labile limit (upper curve) and the maximum equilibrium cholesterol solubility (lower curve).*

the maximum rate of synthesis is approximately 5 g per day.

The gallbladder may sequester almost the entire bile acid pool after an overnight fast. This organ has two important roles: concentration of bile and delivery of bile into the duodenum after food ingestion.[2] Approximately 10% to 30% of the luminal gallbladder volume is absorbed per hour and, given sufficient time, an interprandial reduction of 80% to 90% of the volume of hepatic bile entering the gallbladder can be achieved.[3] The result is a progressive increase in the concentration of bile acids within the lumen.

Filling of the gallbladder is enhanced by the resistance to flow in the duodenum offered by the sphincter of Oddi. The fasting storage pattern of the gallbladder may vary in different subjects, and its regulation is not fully understood. In addition to filling pressure, wall compliance probably helps explain the differences in filling volumes. Also, there are several conditions that increase fasting gallbladder volume. Pregnant women have a resting gallbladder volume nearly twice that of control subjects. This probably results from a combination of decreased water absorption and a diminished tone of the gallbladder wall caused by elevated serum progesterone levels.[4] After total vagotomy, the fasting volume of the gallbladder increased by 15% to 100%, a probable effect of decreased vagal tone.[5]

Gallbladder wall contraction and subsequent emptying after meals is mediated by endogenous release of cholecystokinin (CCK). Ingestion of a standard meal is followed by a prompt rise of the CCK concentration in plasma and subsequent gallbladder emptying. This peak concentration is fivefold greater than the interdigestive level. It appears unlikely that gallbladder contraction is the cause of the delivery, as it is preserved after cholecystectomy.[6]

Whereas the flow of bile down the canaliculi toward the ductules may be facilitated by microtubular contractions, the larger ducts appear to have no functional wall muscle components. Interdigestive flow into the duodenum is determined, then, by biliary secretory pressure, gallbladder compliance, and resistance at the sphincter of Oddi. In addition to causing gallbladder contraction, meal-stimulated release of CCK decreases resistance of the sphincter of Oddi and increases the hepatic secretion of bile.

A pressure profile of the sphincter of Oddi demonstrates a basal pressure that averages 6 mmHg above the common duct pressure. Superimposed on the basal pressure are high-amplitude phasic-wave contractions, which average 4 per minute but have a frequency range as high as 12 per minute. The phasic contractions measure 101 ± 50 mmHg in amplitude and last approximately 4 ± 1.5 seconds.[7]

The exact role of these phasic contraction waves has yet to be defined. However, evidence from several investigators strongly suggests that phasic activity regulates the flow of bile and pancreatic duct contents into the duodenum. Dodds and Toouli have shown that the predominant mechanism for ductal emptying is the antegrade phasic contractions that strip the distal ampulla of its contents. Only small quantities of bile escape into the duodenum prior to the next contraction.[8]

Gallstone Formation

The exact biochemistry of gallstone formation remains elusive. However, in the last two decades, much progress has been made in understanding the probable events.

It is convenient to classify gallstones into two types: cholesterol and pigment. These types are generally easy to distinguish macroscopically and chemically. Cholesterol stones are light brown and smooth or faceted and on cross-section have a laminated or crystalline appearance. Pigment stones are smaller and more numerous, black or brown, irregularly shaped, and amorphous or crystalline on cross-section.[9] The majority of gallstones are not pure but have a mixed chemical composition. Cholesterol-predominant stones, then, make up 70% to 80% of American stones. The following discussion will therefore concentrate on the factors promoting formation of cholesterol stones.

The formation of gallstones depends on at least three factors. First, cholesterol dissolved in bile must be in a supersaturated or unstable state. Second, cholesterol must undergo nucleation to allow it to fall out of solution. Third, the precipitate must persist and allow continued fallout to permit stone growth. Several factors are probably involved in promoting each of these steps to gallstone formation.

Cholesterol Concentration

Cholesterol is virtually insoluble in water. As noted earlier, it is held in solution in bile by its association with the bile salts and phospholipids in the form of mixed micelles (Fig. 1). Early studies confirmed that most gallstone patients secrete a supersaturated bile, leading to an early fixation on this aspect of stone formation.[10] However, cholesterol in mild excess to bile salts and lecithin creates a metastable state and usually precipitates only if there is a promoter to initiate this response. At markedly excessive cholesterol concentrations, true supersaturation occurs, and precipitation then can occur rapidly in the homogeneous solution without initiating factors.

Increased cholesterol saturation could result either from increased cholesterol secretion or from decreased bile salt output. Earlier authors stressed that deficient secretion of bile salts from a contracted pool was the cornerstone of the formation of lithogenic bile.[11] Although this may be true in a few cases, more recent studies suggest that hypersecretion of biliary cholesterol is the principal cause of supersaturation in both obese and nonobese humans in the Western hemisphere.

The cause of the hypersecretion is undoubtedly multifactorial. For example, being female, multiparity, and exogenous estrogen use are all associated with an increased risk of gallstones. Estrogens increase the numbers of hepatocellular binding sites for LDL particles and chylomicron remnants.[12] These lipoproteins deliver the majority of endogenous and exogenous cholesterol to the liver to be utilized or excreted, and this may promote supersaturation even in the face of normal or low serum cholesterol levels. Exogenous obesity also increases the risk of cholelithiasis. Obese patients have increased hepatic and extrahepatic cholesterol synthesis, thus promoting bile saturation.[13] Advancing age also correlates strongly with the risk of carrying gallstones. In fact, in Western men, this is the strongest predictor of stones. This statistic correlates with age-related increments in biliary cholesterol saturation. Decreased hepatic catabolism of cholesterol to bile acids with age has been shown in both sexes in Swedish workers.[14]

Cholesterol is converted to cholesterol esters for storage within the liver. Progestational agents and clofibrate are potent inhibitors of the microsomal enzyme for this conversion, and therapy with these agents thus increases cholesterol secretion and cholesterol saturation of bile.[15] The risk of women in acquiring gallstones increases during the last trimester of pregnancy and may be greater with usage of low-estrogen contraceptive steroid mixtures.[16] Use of clofibrate, a serum lipid-lowering agent, is also associated with an increased risk of gallstone formation.[17]

Prolonged fasting, as during hyperalimentation, is also associated with increased stone formation. In most species, the lipid composition of bile is relatively constant throughout the day; secretion rates of cholesterol and lecithin are proportional to bile acid outputs, and the ratio of cholesterol to lecithin stays relatively constant. In humans, however, this constancy is not maintained. During the day, when the enterohepatic circulation of bile acids is stimulated by food intake, saturation is at its lowest. At night, with fasting, saturation increases. In prolonged fasting, the saturated state may continue indefinitely.[18] This is probably because of the human's inability to reduce cholesterol secretion during fasting to the same extent that bile salt and lecithin secretion is reduced.

Nucleation

Supersaturation is essential for cholesterol gallstone formation, but not everyone with supersaturated bile will form gallstones. Factors favoring crystal formation and growth are also critical to the development of stones. Emphasis has been placed on the difference between the metastable state, in which bile is supersaturated while crystal growth is slow, and the labile state, where the quantity of cholesterol is sufficiently great to crystallize rapidly. However, groups of patients have been studied in whom bile is in the supersaturated state, yet no cholesterol crystals are found. Again, there are probably multiple factors that promote crystallization and growth in stone-forming patients. There appears to be a balance in bile between nucleation inhibitors and promoters and perhaps also between inhibitors and promoters of cholesterol crystal growth. No definite biliary pronucleating or antinucleating proteins or biliary constituents have yet been identified for certain, however.

When the cholesterol content of bile exceeds that which can be solubilized by bile salt and bile salt–lecithin micelles, the excess cholesterol becomes dispersed in much larger lipid vesicles.[19] These vesicles are unilamellar spherical particles composed of a single bilayer of biliary phospholipid (essentially lecithin) and cholesterol. Vesicles are relatively stable and act in concert with micelles as a cholesterol-solubilizing mechanism. It would appear that nucleation of cholesterol crystals occurs only after fusion and aggregation of vesicles to create large liquid crystalline droplets. Once solid cholesterol crystals nucleate, vesicle aggregation does not seem to be repeated.[20] Further crystal growth takes place, not from micelles, but from unilamellar biliary vesicles supersaturated with cholesterol.[21]

In animal models, hypersecretion of mucin glycoproteins by the gallbladder mucosa precedes the clearance of crystalline cholesterol.[22] Mucin glycoprotein gels thus may play an important role in inducing nucleation of crystalline cholesterol. There is evidence that mucin gel hypersecretion may be prostaglandin-mediated. For example, in the prairie dog model, mucin hypersecretion and crystallization can be suppressed by oral aspirin.

Carey proposed that hydrolysis of arachidonyl lecithin by gallbladder mucosa provides the stimulus that induces the prostanoid pathway.[23] Further evidence suggests that hypersecretion of biliary cholesterol is a trigger for hypersecretion of arachidonyl lecithin molecules. Finally, the hepatic secretion of arachidonyl lecithin correlates strongly with secretion of deoxycholic acid. The percentage of biliary deoxycholate has been reported to be consistently higher in the bile of patients with cholesterol gallstones compared with controls.[24]

Gel matrices have long been used in industry to induce nucleation for crystal growth. In the gallbladder, the gel matrix of mucus formed at the wall promotes and supports crystallization by providing the matrix for the initial crystal nucleation from liposomes and further deposition from liquid crystals.[21] Initial aggregation and growth of crystals may also take place on the matrix. This view is supported by the finding of a nidus of mucin glycoproteins with calcium bilirubinate at the center of many cholesterol stones.[25]

Persistence and Growth

Finally, sludge and small stones may be protected from expulsion from the gallbladder by the tenacious mucous coat. This protection may involve promoting increased cystic duct resistance or a direct effect on the wall to decrease contraction.[23] Further stasis would be promoted by factors such as those previously mentioned: prolonged fasting, pregnancy, and vagotomy.

In summary, stone formation is an obviously complex process in which supersaturation of bile to supply cholesterol, crystallization of cholesterol, and stasis without expulsion to promote further growth all must be present. Further understanding of these factors will aid in the selection of appropriate nonsurgical management of stones, the development of methods to deter early recurrence after nonsurgical management, and, perhaps, ultimately in the prevention of stones altogether in some patients.

References

1. Carey MC, Small DM: The physical chemistry of cholesterol solubility in bile. Relationship to gallstone formation and dissolution in man. *J Clin Invest* 1978; 61:998.
2. Paumgartner G, Sauerbruch T: Secretion, composition and flow of bile. *Clin Gastroenterol* 1983; 12:3.
3. Wheeler HO: Concentration function of the gallbladder. *Am J Med* 1971; 51:588.
4. Everson GT, McKinley C, Lawson M, et al: Gallbladder function in the human female: Affect of the ovulary cycle, pregnancy and contraceptive steroids. *Gastroenterology* 1982; 82:711.
5. Kramhoft J, Balslev I, Lindahl F, Backer OG: Vagotomy and function of the gallbladder. *Scand J Gastroenterol* 1972; 7:109.
6. Peeters TL, Vantrappen G, Janssens J: Bile acid output and the interdigestive migrating motor complex in normals and in cholecystectomy patients. *Gastroenterology* 1980; 79:678.
7. Geenen JE, Hogan WJ, Dodds WJ, et al: Intraluminal pressure recording from the human sphincter of Oddi. *Gastroenterology* 1980; 78:317.
8. Toouli J, Honda R, Dodds WJ, et al: Monometric, electric and flow properties of the opossum sphincter of Oddi. *Dig Dis Sci* 1980; 25:719.

9. Boucher IAD: Biochemistry of gallstone formation. *Clin Gastroenterol* 1983; 12:25.

10. Grundy SM, Duane WC, Alder RD, et al: Biliary lipid outputs in young women with cholesterol gallstones. *Metabolism* 1974; 23:67.

11. Shaffer EA, Small DM: Biliary lipid secretion in cholesterol gallstone disease: The effect of cholecystectomy and obesity. *J Clin Invest* 1977; 59:828.

12. Brown MS, Goldstein JL: How LDL receptors influence cholesterol and atherosclerosis. *Sci Am* 1984; 251:58.

13. Bennion LJ, Grundy JM: Effects of obesity and caloric intake on biliary lipid metabolism in man. *J Clin Invest* 1975; 56:996.

14. Einarsson K, Nilsell K, Leijd B, Angelin B: Influence of age on secretion of cholesterol and synthesis of bile acids by the liver. *N Engl J Med* 1985; 313:277.

15. Nervi FO, Del Pozo R, Covarrubias CF, Ronco BO: The effect of progesterone on the regulatory mechanism of biliary cholesterol secretion in the rat. *Hepatology* 1983; 3:360.

16. Down RHL, Whiting ML, Watts JMcK, Jones W: Effect of synthetic estrogens and progestagens in oral contraceptives on bile lipid compositions. *Gut* 1983; 24:253.

17. Grundy SM, Ahrens EM Jr, Salen G, et al: Mechanism of action of clofibrate on cholesterol metabolism in patients with hyperlipidemia. *J Lipid Res* 1972; 13:531.

18. Mok HYI, vonBermann K, Grundy SM: Factors affecting bile saturation at low outputs of bile acids. In: Paumgartner G, Stiehl A, Gerok W (eds): *Biological Effects of Bile Acids,* Freiburg: MPT Press, 1978, p 39.

19. Somjen GJ, Gilat T: A non-micellar mode of cholesterol transport in human bile. *FEBS Lett* 1983; 156:265.

20. Holzbach RT, Corbusier C: Liquid crystals and cholesterol nucleation during equilibrium in supersaturated bile analogs. *Biochim Biophys Acta* 1978; 328:436.

21. Lee SP, Park HZ, Mandan J, Kaler EW: Partial characterization of a non-micellar system of cholesterol solubilization in bile. *Am J Physiol* 1987; 252:G374.

22. Lee SP, LaMont JT, Carey MC: Role of gallbladder mucus hypersecretion in the evolution of cholesterol gallstones: Studies in the prairie dog. *J Clin Invest* 1981; 67:1712.

23. Carey MC, Cahalane MJ: Whither biliary sludge? *Gastroenterology* 1988; 95:508.

24. Carulli N, Loria P, Bertolotti M, et al: Effects of acute changes of bile acid pool composition on biliary lipid secretion. *J Clin Invest* 1985; 74:614.

4

Gallstone Imaging for Extracorporeal Shock Wave Lithotripsy

●

Craig M. Carpenter

Introduction

Prior to the advent of nonsurgical therapy for cholelithiasis, gallstone imaging was a binary decision: are gallstones present or not? Since the introduction of oral bile acid therapy, contact dissolution techniques, and extracorporeal shock wave lithotripsy (ESL), the radiologic evaluation of gallstones has become more complex. Now, the size, number, and radiographic density of gallstones are very important, as they affect the decision about which form of therapy a patient will receive. The functional status of the gallbladder also must be assessed. This complexity has renewed interest in oral cholecystography (OCG). In this chapter, the radiographic evaluation of cholelithiasis as it pertains to ESL will be summarized.

Ultrasonography

Ultrasonography has become the method of choice for the detection of cholelithiasis. Numerous studies comparing the accuracy of high-resolution real-time sonography and OCG have confirmed the former's superior sensitivity.[1,2] Moreover, these studies were performed during the infancy of real-time technology and during a time when the expertise and experience of the sonologist was less extensive. Today, real-time equipment is capable of detecting stones less than 1 mm in diameter.

The sonographic image is created when an electrical current excites a piezoelectric crystal, resulting in the emission of high-frequency sound waves. These sound waves travel through tissues and are reflected from areas of differing acoustic impedance. Transducers emit very rapid pulses of sound and "listen" as the sound waves return from the tissue being interrogated. The sound waves from deeper structures return slightly later than those from more superficial structures. This information is analyzed by a computer and displayed instantaneously as an image on the monitor.

Sound travels easily through fluid-filled structures but is completely reflected by gas and completely attenuated by calcification. These characteristics make ultrasound ideally suited for evaluation of gallstones. Gallstones within the gallbladder appear as echogenic structures that create acoustic shadowing within the normally echo-free bile.

There are a variety of real-time ultrasound units available that have slightly different features and very different price tags. However, all of the units utilize hand-held probes that emit frequencies between 2 and 10 mHz. Higher-frequency probes provide higher resolution, but as the frequency of the transducer increases, the depth of tissue penetration decreases. The frequencies most commonly used for evaluation of the biliary system are 3.5 and 5 mHz; rarely it is necessary to use a 2.0- or 2.25-mHz probe to evaluate obese patients. Because ultrasound does not travel through gas, the probe must be properly coupled to the skin with acoustic gel.

Patients are evaluated in multiple positions during the gallbladder sonogram. One of these must be the left lateral decubitus position because small stones may be obscured in the neck of the gallbladder and become visible only when "rolled out" into the fundus. It is rarely necessary to evaluate patients in the erect position. Multiple transverse and longitudinal images of the gallbladder should be recorded utilizing the highest-frequency transducer capable of penetrating to the required depth. A routine gallbladder sonogram should include evaluation of the bile ducts, contiguous liver, and pancreas.

The number and size of stones should be documented in any patient being considered for nonsurgical therapy. Optimally, stone measurement is performed in the axial (anteroposterior) diameter, because resolution in this dimension is superior to lateral resolution. Axial measurements of larger stones may not be possible, however, as the exact location of the posterior surface of the stone cannot be ascertained because of acoustic shadowing (Fig. 1).

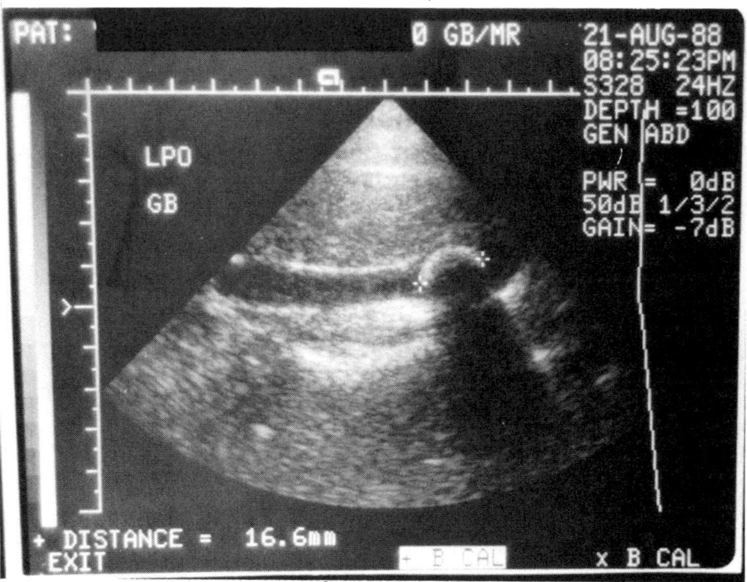

Figure 1: *Left posterior oblique longitudinal image of gallbladder with large 16.6-mm stone. Measurement is made in lateral dimension since true AP (axial) dimensions cannot be ascertained due to acoustic shadowing.*

Therefore, for measuring stones 20 mm or larger, OCG remains more accurate. Images of the stones should be magnified, and cursor readouts of the stone dimensions should be clearly displayed. It is often helpful to obtain hard-copy images of small stones with and without cursor markings, as the cursors often obscure the true margins of small stones within the gallbladder.

Other abnormalities such as contiguous cavernous hemangiomas of the liver, hepatic cysts, and pancreatic pseudocysts should be noted by the radiologist. It is also important to estimate the relation of these structures to the estimated path of the shock waves.

OCG

Since the advent of real-time ultrasound, the number of OCGs has decreased dramatically. In fact, recently trained radiologists often have little experience in performing and interpreting this examination. Since the introduction of ESL in the United States, however, there has been a resurgence of interest in OCG. All cholecystographic agents are administered orally, absorbed by the gastrointestinal tract, excreted into the bile, and passed into the gallbladder via the cystic duct. "Nonvisualization" of the gallbladder may be the result of interference with any of the essential steps of absorption, excretion, or concentration of the agent by the gallbladder (Table 1).

Table 1
Causes of Nonvisualization of the Gallbladder

Gallbladder disease
   Acute cholecystitis (cystic duct obstruction)
   Chronic cholecystitis
   Acalculous cholecystitis
   Cholelithiasis

Liver disease
Malabsorption
Retention of contrast in the esophagus (e.g., stricture) or stomach
Vomiting, diarrhea, or failure to ingest contrast agent

Patients should be evaluated for a history of allergic reactions to radiographic agents prior to oral cholecystography. Those with such an allergy should be premedicated with corticosteroids, as cross-reactions do occur. Because renal failure has been described in patients receiving high-dose OCG examinations, routine use of double-dose examinations should be avoided. The patient should not be dehydrated during the examination, because these agents have powerful uricosuric affects.

The two most common agents utilized for OCG are Telepaque and Oragrafin. Telepaque is a fat-soluble compound that requires concomitant fat ingestion for maximum absorption. Maximum gallbladder opacification occurs 14 to 16 hours later. Oragrafin is a water-soluble compound and therefore may be administered without a fatty meal. Maximum gallbladder opacification occurs 6 to 8 hours after administration.

Ideally, a preliminary film of the gallbladder is obtained prior to the administration of contrast material to avoid obscuration of calcified stones by the contrast agent. Multiple supine and erect spot films of the gallbladder utilizing graded compression and oblique filming are usually sufficient to diagnose calcified stones in the fundus of an opacified gallbladder. Because most ESL protocols exclude stones that contain calcium, right upper-quadrant radiographs are obtained at some point in the pre-ESL evaluation. These films should ideally be performed with the patient prone and should be "coned down" to the right upper quadrant (Fig. 2). Calcification is best seen on low-kVp, high-mA films.

Sonographic–Cholecystographic Correlation

The OCG had been the gold standard for diagnosis of cholelithiasis for approximately 50 years prior to sonography. Soon after the inception of ultrasonography, the OCG became almost obsolete in clinical practice. Sonography has proved to be far more sensitive for the detection of small stones, does not involve ionizing radiation, requires no con-

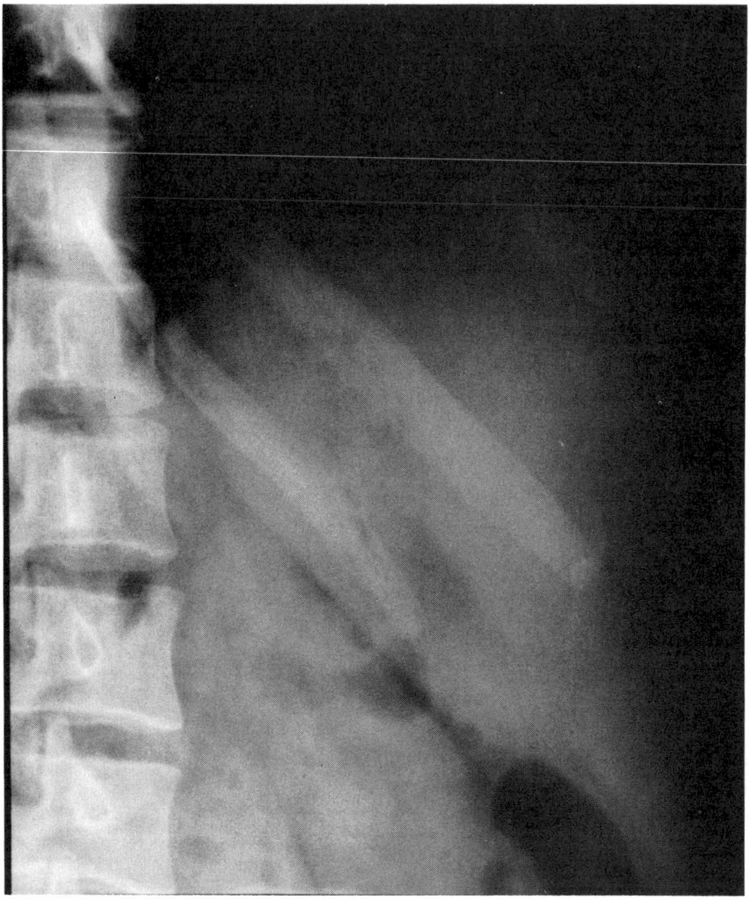

Figure 2: *Coned-down view of the right upper quadrant (prone position) is more effective than coned down view of the right upper quadrant in supine position or "KUB" film in detecting calcification. No calcification seen in the gallstones in this patient.*

trast material, allows a survey of other abdominal structures, and may be performed on an emergency basis. However, ultrasound is less consistently accurate in defining the exact number of gallstones than is OCG. Also, OCG permits more precise measurements of larger stones and better illustrates the stone contour, especially in the case of nonspherical stones. Evaluation of stones in multiple projections by ultrasound and OCG is usually necessary to depict exactly the size, number, and shape of gallstones.

Patient Eligibility for ESL

Candidates for nonsurgical therapy must have a functioning gallbladder on OCG. In a survey of asymptomatic patients in Italy with sonographically proved cholelithiasis, there was 28% incidence of nonvisualization on OCG.[3] A slightly higher rate of nonvisualization is to be expected in symptomatic individuals.

The Italian study also demonstrated an 18% incidence of radiographically evident calcification of gallstones. A recent study at Massachusetts General Hospital showed that 17% of 100 consecutive surgically removed gallbladders contained calcified gallstones.[4] It was also noted that 63% of gallbladders contained more than three stones. The conclusion was that approximately 15% of patients with cholelithiasis are candidates for ESL under the current criteria. This has been the experience at our institution and at other institutions screening patients for ESL.

Imaging for ESL

The patient should undergo ultrasound of the gallbladder just prior to induction of anesthesia to ensure that the stones are still present and to document the size of the common bile duct. The position of the gallbladder should then be marked on the patient's skin. If the procedure is to be performed with the patient prone, the gallbladder position should also be marked on the patient's side in the anterior or midaxillary line. In very obese patients, the gallbladder should be scanned in the prone position prior to anesthesia to assure adequate imaging during the procedure.

Once ESL is begun, real-time sonographic evaluation should be performed to monitor the procedure (Fig. 3A-F). Movement of the stones with each shock wave or swirling of bile from the gallbladder usually is seen. If not, the stones should be relocalized before continuing therapy. As frag-

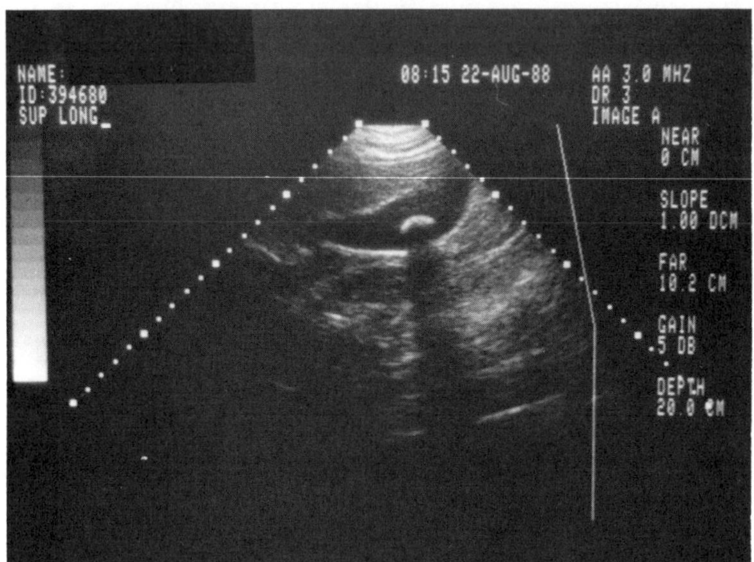

Figure 3: *A. Supinal longitudinal image of gallbladder immediately prior to lithotripsy.*

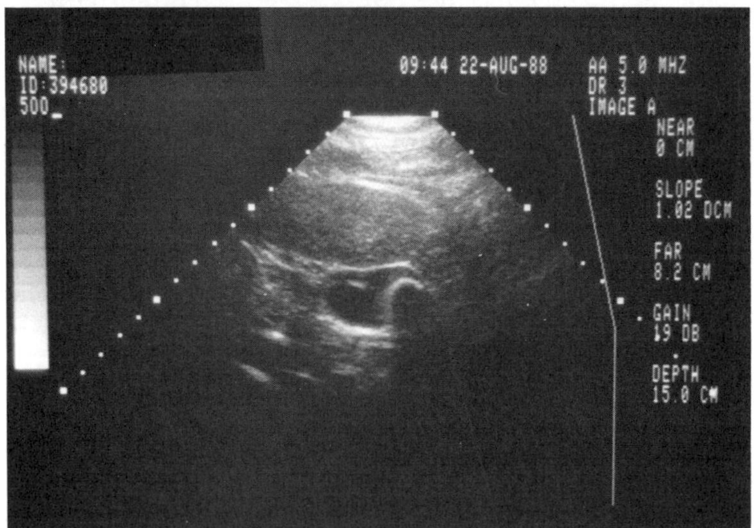

Figure 3: *B. Following 500 shock waves, there is partial fragmentation of the stone. The large fragment still resides in the fundus of the gallbladder, but a smaller fragment is noted in the neck.*

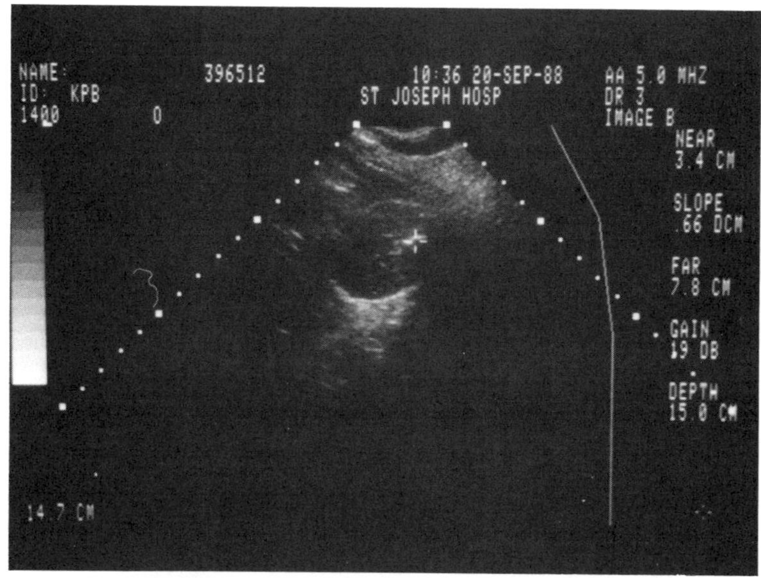

Figure 3: *C. Following 1,400 shocks, there are multiple small fragments, the largest fragment measuring approximately 5 mm in diameter.*

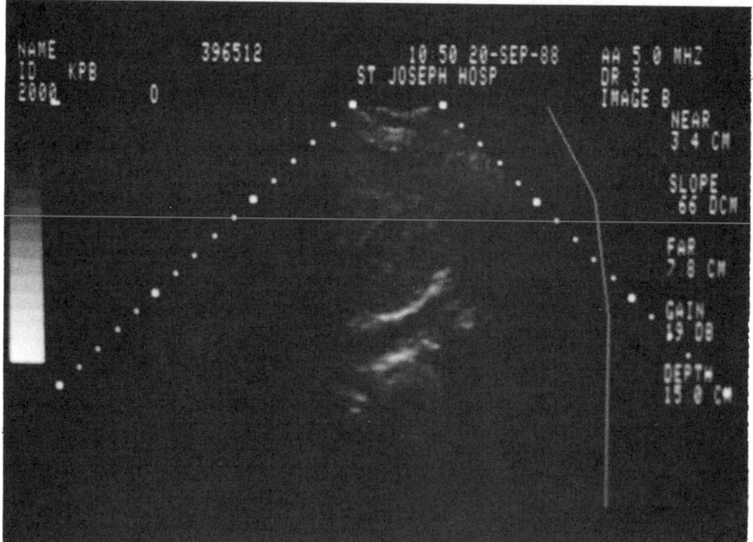

Figure 3: *D. Following 2,000 shocks, the gallbladder contains multiple small fragments, less than 2 mm in size.*

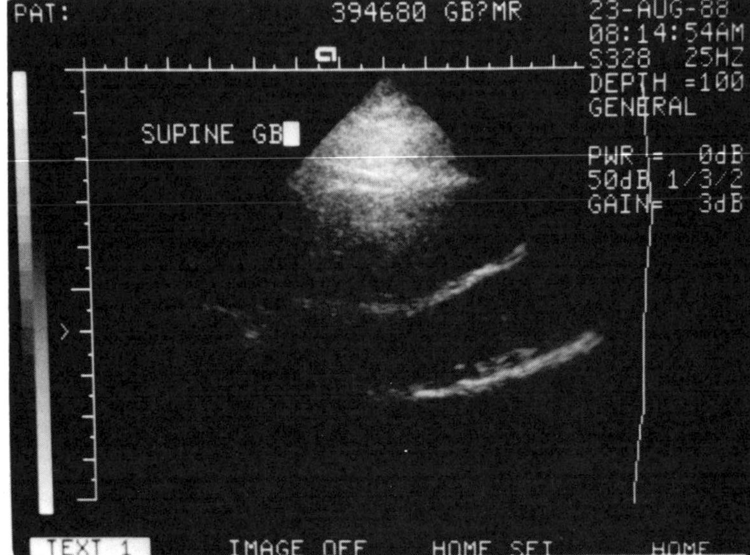

Figure 3: *E. One month following lithotripsy, there are multiple small fragments within the gallbladder.*

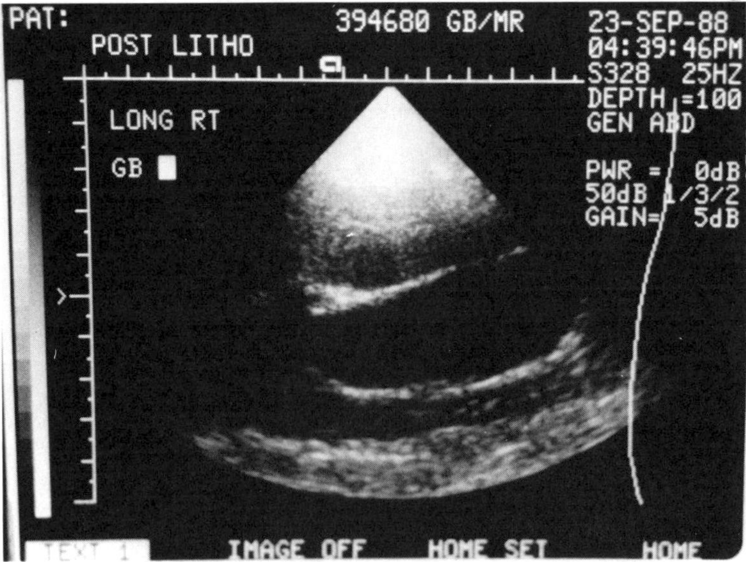

Figure 3: *F. Two months following lithotripsy, a very few minute fragments remain within the gallbladder. Subsequent sonograms on this patient were normal.*

mentation of the stone proceeds, a "cloud" of small fragments is usually visible. This cloud may partially obscure larger fragments within the gallbladder. Frequent careful examination of the gallbladder should be performed to document the position of the largest fragments. The procedure should be terminated when the largest residual fragments are no larger than 4 mm.

Follow-up sonograms are usually obtained in 24 hours and then at monthly intervals as needed. Careful attention to the number and size of fragments is very important. Complications such as bile duct dilation, pancreatitis, or abnormalities of the gallbladder wall should be noted. Because the fragments may be small, it is very important to evaluate patients in multiple positions to ensure that small fragments are not hidden in the neck or the proximal cystic duct.

Conclusion

The radiographic evaluation of gallstones has become more complex in the era of ESL. The exact number, size, and morphology of gallstones should be documented as thoroughly as possible on all routine gallbladder ultrasound studies. Oral cholecystography and plain radiography performed on patients who are potentially candidates should be carefully correlated in order to screen patients optimally for ESL. As selection criteria are broadened, these data will become essential in predicting the efficacy of ESL in individual patients.

References

1. Krook PM, Allen FH, Bush WJ Jr, et al: Comparison of real-time cholecystosonography and oral cholecystography. *Radiology* 1980; 35:145.
2. deGraff CS, Denbner AG, Taylor KJW: Ultrasound and false normal oral cholecystogram. *Arch Surg* 1978; 113:877.
3. Rome Group for Epidemiology and Prevention of Cholelithiasis (GREPCO): Radiology appearance of gallstones and its relationship with biliary symptoms and awareness of hav-

ing gallstones: Observations during epidemiological studies. *Dig Dis Sci* 1987; 32:349.
4. Brink JA, Simeone JF, Mueller PR, et al: Physical characteristics of gallstones removed at cholecystectomy: Implications for extracorporeal shock wave lithotripsy. *AJR* 1988; 151:927.

5

Overview of Gallstone Management

Daniel H. Dunn

Introduction

The management of patients who have biliary tract disease has evolved from a period when oral and intravenous cholangiography and cholecystectomy and common bile duct exploration were the only diagnostic and therapeutic measures available. Today, multiple invasive and noninvasive diagnostic techniques are being utilized, and nonsurgical treatment of biliary tract disease, both calculus and noncalculus, is commonplace. This chapter discusses the currently accepted surgical and nonsurgical approaches to the treatment of calculus biliary disease.

Changing Attitudes Toward Management

In the 1960s, operating on asymptomatic patients was common because of studies showing that 50% of those patients developed biliary colic or complications from gallstones.[1,2] However, these studies included only patients who had already had at least one episode of biliary colic; subsequent studies of truly asymptomatic patients followed for as long as 24 years showed that symptoms develop at a rate of approximately 2% per year.[3-5] Importantly, complications of gallstones were almost always preceded by biliary symptoms, refuting the argument that prophylactic cholecystectomy was warranted to prevent complications of cholelithiasis as the initial presentation of biliary tract disease.

Surgeons have been quick to point out that the operative mortality rate for elective cholecystectomy is extremely low, whereas when patients reach 65 years of age, the operative mortality rate increases to 3% to 10%, and that in patients operated on after presenting with complications such as cholangitis, the mortality rate is even higher, the contention being that early cholecystectomy would avert these complications and minimize the mortality rate. However, subsequent studies showed that cholecystectomy in asymptomatic patients would actually reduce the overall life expectancy.[6] Moreover, the costs of "prophylactic" cholecystectomies in the asymptomatic population would be tremendous. Therefore, the exclusion of asymptomatic patients from either medical or surgical treatment seems to be justified. This is true even in diabetic patients, as there is little evidence that these patients are more likely to suffer complications.[7,8]

Management of Chronic Cholecystitis

Once the diagnosis of chronic cholecystitis has been established and the patient and physician agree that the symptoms are severe enough to warrant treatment, cholecystectomy has been the traditional recommendation. Now, with the introduction of oral and percutaneous dissolution therapy and, most recently, biliary lithotripsy, nonsurgical therapy for gallstones will likely become more important.

Surgery

The success of cholecystectomy for the treatment of gallbladder stones is attributable to several factors. First, it relieves the symptoms in all but a few patients, even if the symptoms are atypical. Second, there is no chance for recurrent stones because the gallbladder has been removed.

An earlier problem, namely stones left in the common bile duct, now can generally be managed by endoscopic retrograde cholangiopancreatoscopy (ERCP) and sphincterotomy, so reoperative surgery for retained stones is now a rarity. Third, the operative mortality rate is less than 0.3% in patients with uncomplicated biliary tract disease who are under 50 years of age, and the morbidity is equally low. The higher mortality rate quoted in some studies is attributable largely to the inclusion of patients who are elderly or who have complications of cholelithiasis, such as acute cholecystitis, cholangitis, and common bile duct stones.

Despite this success, patients obviously would like to avoid surgery, and the postoperative recovery period, the 4 to 6 weeks away from work, the surgical scar, and the possible postoperative complications have kept many symptomatic patients from seeking medical and surgical care. In the search for an effective, safe nonsurgical method for ridding the gallbladder of stones, various dissolving agents, such as chenodeoxycholic acid (CDCA), ursodeoxycholic acid (UDCA), monooctanoin, and methyl tert-butyl ether, have been subjected to clinical trials.

Dissolution Therapy

Oral

Ursodeoxycholate is a secondary bile acid which is a 7β epimer of CDCA. Both agents have been given orally to dissolve small noncalcified, floating radiolucent gallstones.[9,10] The rate of complete dissolution of stones, 13% to 25% in a selected subgroup of patients over 1.5 to 2 years of treatment, makes it difficult to recommend this treatment modality. The side effects of CDCA (hepatic toxicity and diarrhea) and the 10% per year gallstone recurrence rate are additional drawbacks. Ursodeoxycholic acid, which has just been approved for general use in the United States, has no reported hepatotoxicity and a very low incidence of diarrhea. The chief role of UDCA may be in combination with biliary lithotripsy. The reports of such treatment from Europe have been encouraging, and are ongoing in the United States.

Percutaneous

It would seem logical that stone dissolution would be more effective if the stones were bathed directly in a solvent. Numerous attempts to do this with agents such as diethyl ether and chloroform infused via a T-tube placed intraoperatively produced significant side effects and low success rates.[11,12] More recently, however, two agents—monooctanoin and methyl tert-butyl ether (MTBE)—have been successful in many patients with fewer side effects. This treatment has been especially useful when combined with interventional radiologic techniques that gain access to the biliary tract without open operation.

Monooctanoin is a medium-chain diglyceride that solubilizes cholesterol. There is a correlation between the percentage of cholesterol in the stones and the success rate. MTBE, a less-explosive analog of diethyl ether, works faster than monooctanoin in many cases, although some stones that will not dissolve in MTBE will dissolve in monooctanoin. MTBE can be used only for stones in the gallbladder because of the side effects produced by the solvent in the common duct or duodenum. Special precautions are necessary for its safe handling.

Both monooctanoin and MTBE are often used together with mechanical extraction or fragmentation techniques to reduce further the time needed to rid the patient of stones. These uses have recently been reviewed.[13,14]

Management of Acute Cholecystitis

The management of acute cholecystitis has certainly changed over the past 15 years. Formerly, the initial treatment for acute, uncomplicated cholecystitis was nonoperative, with patients given nothing by mouth and receiving intravenous fluid and antibiotics. If the patients improved, they were discharged to return in 6 to 8 weeks for elective cholecystectomy.

Unfortunately, many patients became sicker while being observed and had to be operated on under less than ideal conditions. Additionally, those who recovered during several days in the hospital had to be hospitalized again for a similar period to recover from the cholecystectomy. Also, some patients did not come back for cholecystectomy, returning only with another episode of cholecystitis. Still others would have an exacerbation of the cholecystitis while waiting to have their cholecystectomy. Thus, surgeons began to recommend early cholecystectomy, within 24 to 48 hours after admission following initial resuscitation. Several controlled trials confirmed the wisdom of early operation, for the mortality rate was lower, the incidence of complications was similar in the two groups, the total length of hospital stay was markedly reduced, and the total cost was less in those patients who had immediate cholecystectomy.[15-18] In those patients who are particularly ill and have little reserve to tolerate complications, early operation is especially warranted.[19,20]

Management of Acute Cholangitis

Charcot's initial description in 1877 of fever and chills, abdominal pain, and jaundice elucidated a clinical entity that was associated with a high mortality rate.[21] In 1959, Reynolds and Dargan added mental confusion and shock as two signs of particularly poor prognosis in patients with suppurative cholangitis.[22]

Extensive clinical research has shown that two conditions must exist for this clinical syndrome to manifest itself. First, the bile must have bacteria in significant numbers, and, second, there must be at least partial obstruction of the biliary tract to cause an increase in biliary ductal pressure leading to biliary venous reflux. Although strictures and carcinoma have been associated with cholangitis, the majority of patients have common bile duct stones.

Surgical decompression of the biliary tract has been the standard to which all other treatments are compared. The first line of treatment is aggressive use of broad-spectrum antibiotics. Because the bacteria most commonly isolated from the bile of patients with cholangitis are *E. coli, Klebsiella pneumoniae,* enterococci, and *Bacteroides,* the antibiotics chosen should be effective against these organisms. An aminoglycoside, ampicillin and metronidazole, or clindamycin will be effective against most organisms from the gastrointestinal tract. Triple antibiotic therapy covering gram-negatives, gram-positives, and anaerobes has been the gold standard but has been challenged recently by single-drug therapy with third-generation cephalosporins.[23] Nevertheless, many surgeons are hesitant to abandon a drug regimen that has proved so effective.

Once the patient has been resuscitated and stabilized and antibiotics have been given, the second step is decompression of the biliary tract, which can be accomplished by operation, endoscopic sphincterotomy, or percutaneous transhepatic drainage (PTD).

The primary goal of surgery is to provide drainage of the common bile duct as quickly and safely as possible. The common bile duct may be opened initially, the common duct stones removed, and a T-tube placed for drainage. Flushing or extensive manipulation of the bile duct in a patient with septic cholangitis is ill advised. A cholecystectomy must also be performed if the patient has concomitant acute cholecystitis. However, most patients are stable enough that a formal common bile duct exploration can be performed, with cholangiography before and after duct exploration. A cholecystectomy is performed at the same time. All patients who do not require immediate operative treatment should have a thorough evaluation, including ERCP or percutaneous transhepatic cholangiogram (PTC), prior to surgical exploration, as undetected biliary strictures, abscesses, or stones may go untreated if not delineated preoperatively and may increase the morbidity or mortality.[24] Evaluation should be carried out only when the patient no longer has signs of cholangitis.

Prior to the advent of PTC and PTD and of ERCP and sphincterotomy, surgical decompression of the biliary tract was the only definitive treatment. However, patients who presented with septic shock had a very high mortality rate, in the range of 50%, and if these patients did not have emergency surgical decompression, the mortality rate was even higher. Although the mortality rates have declined, the basic principles of management remain the same.

New techniques for biliary drainage have been made available. Percutaneous transhepatic drainage for acute cholangitis was first reported more than 10 years ago.[25] Since then, other series have documented the value of this alternative to surgical decompression[26] with especially impressive results considering that patients treated with PTD probably were less stable than those who were operated on. This procedure does require special expertise, and the interventional radiologist must be experienced to keep the morbidity and mortality rates low.

ERCP has largely replaced PTC as a diagnostic tool in patients with biliary tract disease, just as endoscopic sphincterotomy is displacing PTD as a technique to drain the biliary tract. However, unlike operative decompression of the common bile duct, the success of sphincterotomy is very operator-dependent, and few gastroenterologists have the experience and the expertise to perform this procedure safely, effectively, and reliably. A few reports suggest that the mortality rate of sphincterotomy is similar to that of common bile duct exploration in patients with acute cholangitis.[27] This statistic may be attributable to the severe nature of the underlying disease process, namely sepsis, or to the fact that the selection process would move the sicker patients to sphincterotomy rather than operation. Only time and a greater experience will determine the final role of PTD, endoscopic sphincterotomy, and surgical drainage in patients with acute cholangitis.

Management of Biliary Pancreatitis

In 1900, Opie described the pathological association of pancreatitis and choledocholithiasis in a patient who died of acute necrotizing pancreatitis with a stone impacted in the ampulla of Vater.[28] He hypothesized that bile reflux into the pancreatic duct caused pancreatitis and thus originated the common channel theory. Subsequent studies challenged this theory, as pancreatic ductal pressure is usually higher than biliary pressure, which should prevent reflux. However, more recent studies have again established the importance of a stone passing through or impacted in the ampulla as the causative factor in biliary pancreatitis.[29-31] For example, in one study, 75% of the patients operated on for biliary pancreatitis within 24 hours of onset of symptoms had ampullary stones.[31] Acosta and Ledesma found gallstones in the stools of 34 of 36 patients who had gallstone pancreatitis.[29] Further studies also have revealed predisposing factors that may contribute to the development of gallstone pancreatitis, namely, cystic duct diameter in relation to the size and configuration of the gallstones.[32]

The initial treatment for patients suspected of having gallstone pancreatitis is similar to that of patients who have pancreatitis from other causes. The patient should not take anything by mouth, fluid resuscitation should include crystalloid as well as colloid, blood should be replaced as necessary, and calcium and other electrolytes should be carefully monitored in the early phase of the disease. Parenteral nutrition may be necessary if the pancreatitis does not resolve in 4 to 5 days. In addition, broad-spectrum antibiotics should be given to patients with gallstone pancreatitis, because the incidence of septic complications is higher than in those patients with alcoholic or idiopathic pancreatitis.[31]

If a patient's condition deteriorates in the first 24 to 48 hours, consideration should be given to early operation, which should include cholecystectomy and common bile duct exploration if a stone is demonstrated on cholangiography and sphincteroplasty if the stone is impacted in the ampulla. Although traditional wisdom was that to operate on patients with pancreatitis was lethal, recent studies have shown that operation can be accomplished with a relatively low mortality rate.[33] However, others disagree; in fact, Ranson reported a 65% mortality rate in patients who had early operation (less than 48 hours after onset of symptoms) versus an 18% rate in those patients operated on after pancreatitis resolved.[34] Other reports likewise demonstrated a much higher mortality rate with early than with delayed operation.[35,36] In a prospective study, 70 patients with gallstone pancreatitis were randomized to either operation within 72 hours or to conventional treatment with operation 3 months later.[30] One patient in the early-operation group and two patients in the other group died. The reason the mortality rate was so low in this study was probably the relatively mild pancreatitis in this group of patients.

In summary, operations on the biliary tract may be performed early in the course of gallstone pancreatitis if the patient has mild pancreatitis or if the patient is rapidly deteriorating and there is concern that a stone is impacted in the ampulla of Vater.

An option that has become available recently for patients in the acute phase of gallstone pancreatitis is endoscopic sphincterotomy. In 1981, Safrany and Cotton reported excellent results with early ERCP and sphincterotomy.[37] Other reports have supported the concept of early intervention in patients with worsening pancreatitis, showing low mortality rates under these circumstances.[38,39] Because patients will improve rapidly after sphincterotomy, this treatment should be considered if an experienced endoscopist is available. Whether endoscopic sphincterotomy should be performed electively depends largely on whether the gallbladder has been removed previously. If the gallbladder is absent, then the procedure of choice would be ERCP and sphincterotomy. If the gallbladder is present and the patient is a good operative candidate, then cholecystectomy and common duct exploration should be performed. If the patient is a prohibitive operative risk and the gallbladder is present, consideration should still be given to performing ERCP and sphincterotomy if common duct stones are present.

Because most patients improve after the onset of symptoms of gallstone pancreatitis, operative or endoscopic intervention is not necessary as an emergency procedure. Once the pancreatitis resolves, an elective procedure can be performed. Whether this should be done on the same hospitalization or 6 weeks later has been the subject of considerable controversy, but most authors now agree that early operation, when pancreatitis has resolved, has the same mortality and morbidity rates but with a shorter total hospital stay and therefore more rapid recovery than delayed operation.[40-42] The rationale for early operation is that 25% to 56% of patients with an episode of gallstone pancreatitis will have a recurrent attack within 3 months if the biliary tract pathology is not corrected.[43] Thus, operation early after the resolution of the initial attack of gallstone pancreatitis will prevent further episodes and will avert a second hospitalization and a second recovery period.

Conclusion

Clearly, the therapeutic options for treatment of calculous biliary tract disease have multiplied in the past decade. In addition to the methods mentioned here, there are extracorporeal shock wave lithotripsy, discussed in detail by other contributors to this volume, and percutaneous lithotripsy, including that by laser.[44]

References

1. Lund J: Surgical indications in cholelithiasis: Prophylactic cholecystectomy elucidated on the basis of long-term follow-up on 526 nonoperated cases. *Ann Surg* 1960; 151:153.
2. Wenckert A, Robertson B: The natural course of gallstone disease: Eleven-year review of 781 non-operated cases. *Gastroenterology* 1966; 50:376.
3. Gracie WA, Ransohoff DF: The natural history of silent gallstones: The innocent gallstone is not a myth. *N Engl J Med* 1982; 307:798.
4. McSherry CK, Ferstenberg H, Calhoun WF, et al: The natural history of diagnosed gallstone disease in symptomatic and asymptomatic patients. *Ann Surg* 1985; 202:59.
5. Thistle JL, Cleary PA, Lachin JM, et al: The natural history of cholelithiasis: The National Cooperative Gallstone Study. *Ann Intern Med* 1984; 101:171.
6. Ransohoff DF, Gracie WA, Wolfenson LB, et al: Prophylactic cholecystectomy or expectant management for silent gallstones. *Ann Intern Med* 1983; 99:199.
7. Walsh DB, Eckhauser FE, Ramsburgh SR, et al: Risk associated with diabetes mellitus in patients undergoing gallbladder surgery. *Surgery* 1982; 91:254.
8. Sandler RS, Maule WF, Baltus ME: Factors associated with

postoperative complications in diabetes following biliary tract surgery. *Gastroenterology* 1986; 91:157.

 9. Nakayama F: Oral cholelitholysis: Cheno versus urso. Japanese experience. *Dig Dis Sci* 1980; 25:129.
10. Schoenfield LJ, Lachin JM, et al: Chenodiol (chenodeoxycholic acid) for dissolution of gallstones: The National Cooperative Gallstone Study. *Ann Intern Med* 1981; 95:257.
11. Strickler JH, Adkins DC, Rice CO: Ether flush treatment of retained postoperative common duct stones. *Minn Med* 1954; 37:490.
12. Sasson L: Dissolution and flushing techniques for removal of retained common bile duct stones. *Am J Gastroenterol* 1969; 51:394.
13. Bender CE, Williams HJ: Technical aspects of percutaneous gallstone dissolution. *Semin Intervent Radiol* 1988; 5 (in press).
14. Brandon JC, Teplick SK: New approaches to common bile duct calculi: Roles of methyl *tert*-butyl ether, mono-octanoin, and mechanical fragmentation. *Semin Intervent Radiol* 1988; 5 (in press).
15. van der Linden W, Sunzel H: Early versus delayed operation for acute cholecystitis: A controlled clinical trial. *Am J Surg* 1970; 120:7.
16. McArthur P, Cuschieri A, Sells RA, Shields R: Controlled clinical trial comparing early with interval cholecystectomy for acute cholecystitis. *Br J Surg* 1975; 62:850.
17. Lahtinen I, Alhava EM, Auke S: Acute cholecystitis treated by early and delayed surgery: A controlled clinical trail. *Scand J Gastroenterol* 1978; 13:673.
18. Jarvinen JH, Hastbacka J: Early cholecystectomy for acute cholecystitis: A prospective randomized study. *Ann Surg* 1980; 191:501.
19. Morrow DJ, Thompson J, Wilson SE: Acute cholecystitis in the elderly: A surgical emergency. *Arch Surg* 1978; 113:1149.
20. Houghton PWJ, Jenkinson LR, Donaldson LA: Cholecystectomy in the elderly: A prospective study. *Br J Surg* 1985; 72:220.
21. Charcot JM: Leçons sur les maladies du foie des voies biliaires et des veins. Paris, Bourneville et Sevestre, 1877.
22. Reynolds BM, Dargan EL: Acute obstructive cholangitis: A distinct clinical syndrome. *Ann Surg* 1959; 150:299.
23. Jensen LS, Anderson F, Gjode P, et al: Peroperative cefuroxine vs. long-term ampicillin and metronidazole in high risk biliary and gastric surgery: A multicentre trial. *Acta Chir Scand* 1987; 153:193.

24. Saharia PC, Cameron JL: Clinical management of cholangitis. *Surg Gynecol Obstet* 1976; 142:369.
25. Nakayama T, Ikeda A, Okuda K: Percutaneous transhepatic drainage of the biliary tract: Technique and results in 104 cases. *Gastroenterology* 1978; 74:554.
26. Kadir S, Baassiri A, Barth KH, et al: Percutaneous biliary drainage in the management of biliary sepsis. *Am J Roentgenol* 1982; 138:25.
27. Siegel JH: Endoscopic papillotomy in the treatment of biliary tract disease: 258 procedures and results. *Dig Dis Sci* 1981; 26:1057.
28. Opie EL: The etiology of acute hemorrhagic pancreatitis. *Johns Hopkins Bull* 1901; 121:182.
29. Acosta JM, Ledesma CL: Gallstone migration as a cause of acute pancreatitis. *N Engl J Med* 1974; 290:484.
30. Stone HH, Fabian TC, Dunlop WE: Gallstone pancreatitis: biliary tract pathology in relation to time of operation. *Ann Surg* 1981; 194:305.
31. Acosta JM, Pellegrini CA, Skinner DB: Etiology and pathogenesis of acute biliary pancreatitis. *Surgery* 1980; 88:118.
32. McMahon MJ, Shefta JR: Physical characteristics of gallstones and the calibre of the cystic duct in patients with acute pancreatitis. *Br J Surg* 1980; 67:6.
33. Acosta JM, Rossi R, Galli MR, et al: Early surgery for acute gallstone pancreatitis: Evaluation of a systematic approach. *Surgery* 1978; 83:367.
34. Ranson JHC: Conservative surgical treatment of acute pancreatitis. *World J Surg* 1981; 5:351.
35. Kelly TR: Gallstone pancreatitis: The timing of surgery. *Surgery* 1980; 88:345.
36. Ranson JHC: The timing of biliary surgery in acute pancreatitis. *Ann Surg* 1979; 189:654.
37. Safrany L, Cotton PB: A preliminary report: Urgent duodenoscopic sphincterectomy for acute gallstone pancreatitis. *Surgery* 1981; 89:424.
38. Roesch W, Demling I: Endoscopic management of pancreatitis. *Surg Clin North Am* 1982; 62:845.
39. van der Spuy S: Endoscopic sphincterotomy in the management of gallstone pancreatitis. *Endoscopy* 1981; 13:25.
40. Kim U, Sheth M: Optimal timing of surgical intervention in patients with acute pancreatitis associated with cholelithiasis. *Surg Gynecol Obstet* 1980; 150:499.
41. Paloyan D, Simonowitz D, Skinner DB: The timing of biliary

tract operations in patients with pancreatitis associated with gallstones. *Surg Gynecol Obstet* 1975; 141:737.

42. Elfström J: The timing of cholecystectomy in patients with gallstone pancreatitis. *Acta Chir Scand* 1978; 144:487.
43. Satiani R, Stone HH: Predictability of present outcome and future recurrence in acute pancreatitis. *Arch Surg* 1979; 114:711.
44. Nishioka NS: Laser lithotripsy of biliary calculi. *Semin Intervent Radiol* 1988; 5 (in press).

6

Biliary Lithotripsy

●

Ronald C. Jones, David Vanderpool,
J. Patrick O'Leary, and J. Kent Hamilton

Disease is very old, and nothing about it has changed.
It is we who change, as we recognize what was formerly
imperceptible.

—Charcot

Introduction

It is estimated that 25 million patients in the United States have cholelithiasis, which represents approximately 10% of the population.[1] Gallstones are the most common indication for abdominal surgery, accounting for more than 500,000 operations annually in the United States.[2]

Cholesterol stones constitute 80% of the stones found in Americans, although only about 10% of these are pure cholesterol. Rather, most stones are of mixed composition consisting of more than 70% cholesterol plus calcium, bile acids and pigments, fatty acids, proteins, and phospholipids. The remaining 20% of gallstones are composed primarily of calcium bilirubinate with less than 10% cholesterol.[3]

The first cholecystectomy was performed more than 100 years ago in 1882 by Langebuch,[4] and it has since become a safe and effective treatment for cholelithiasis. Nevertheless, it is a major operation, and in recent years, nonoperative alternatives have been sought. The use of or-

71

ally administered bile acids for the dissolution of gallstones has been disappointing because it is slow, expensive, and often ineffective.[5,6] Percutaneous or endoscopic retrograde instillation of solvents into the biliary tree appears to be successful, but it necessitates invasive intubation of the biliary tract and has been associated with significant complications. These treatments are discussed by Dunn in Chapter 5.

Development of Extracorporeal Lithotripsy

Extracorporeal shock wave lithotripsy (ESL) was first used in humans in 1980, at the Klinikum Grosshadern in Munich, to break up renal calculi.[7] In 1983, Brendel and Enders reported fragmentation of human gallstones implanted in the gallbladders of dogs by lithotripsy,[8] and in 1986, Sauerbruch and associates reported successful ESL for gallstones in 14 patients, nine with stones in the gallbladder and five with stones in the common bile duct.[9] The patients were immersed in water under general anesthesia, and 600 to 1,500 shock waves, synchronized with the electrocardiogram, were delivered. The five patients with common duct stones underwent a sphincterotomy, and a nasobiliary catheter was placed, permitting injection of contrast medium for imaging of the common bile duct and the stones. The gallbladder patients received a combination of ursodeoxycholic acid and chenodeoxycholic acid, both at 7 to 8 mg/kg of body weight per day, to dissolve stone fragments that did not pass spontaneously into the intestine. The bile salts were started 1 week before the shock wave application and continued for as long as 6 months after complete disappearance of stones. Among the patients with gallstones, the six with solitary stones 22 mm or less had complete disappearance of their calculi. However, the three patients with two or three stones had persistence of fragments during the follow-up period (up to 34 weeks). One of the patients had mild pancreatitis. Two of five patients who underwent endoscopic sphincterotomy required basket extraction of their stones. Sauerbruch and associates estimated that only about

5% to 10% of the entire population of patients with gallbladder or common-duct stones referred to their hospital were suitable candidates for ESL.[9]

Sackmann and associates from the Ludwig Maximilian University of Munich reported the first ten patients treated with shock waves without general anesthesia in 1987.[10] Patients were partially immersed in the water bath of the gallstone lithotriptor in a prone position and had to lie still and hold their breath for 5- to 10-second periods to minimize movement of the stones during shock-wave application. Pain was reasonably well tolerated with the administration of analgesics.

In 1988, the first patient in the United States was treated successfully in a completely noninvasive manner with a combination of ESL and bile acid therapy under a Food and Drug Administration (FDA)-approved protocol, at Baylor University Medical Center (BUMC) in Dallas by the authors, using a Medstone 1050 unit. In this chapter, we summarize our experience to date.

Patient Selection

As in any procedure, the results are often dependent on careful patient selection. Rather rigid criteria have been established by the FDA Device Division in approving biliary lithotripsy as an investigational procedure. These criteria, which are based on empiricism as well as on the results from the published European experience, can be divided into two types: those for inclusion and those for exclusion (Table 1).

Prior to being included in the BUMC study cohort, all patients underwent screening procedures that included a thorough medical history, physical examination including stool guaiac, complete blood cell and platelet count, clinical chemistry screen (AST, ALT, creatinine phosphokinase, alkaline phosphatase, total bilirubin, blood urea nitrogen, and creatinine), clotting tests (prothrombin time, partial thromboplastin time, bleeding time), urinalysis, electrocardiogram (to identify any irregular sinus rhythm), chest roentgenogram, oral cholecystogram, ultrasonic imaging of the gall-

Table 1
Patient Selection for ESL

Inclusion Criteria
    History of biliary colic
    Age 18–75 years
    One or more radiolucent gallbladder stones, the largest with a
        diameter between 4 and 20 mm*
    Gallbladder opacification on oral cholecystography
    Shock wave path that avoids lungs and bone
    Written informed consent

Exclusion Criteria
    Acute cholecystitis, pancreatitis, cholangitis, biliary obstruction
        bile-duct stone, or significant liver disease
    Gastroduodenal ulcers that investigator feels may increase risk to
        patient
    Current medication with anticoagulants, aspirin, or nonsteroidal
        antiinflammatory drugs
    Pregnancy
    Gallstone calcification of any extent or distribution as determined
        by cone-down-view x-ray
    Allergy to contrast agents, iodine, bile acids, or lactose
    AST or ALT outside the normal range by more than 20% not
        secondary to gallstone disease
    Presence of cardiac pacemaker
    Bleeding disorders as determined by PT, PTT, bleeding time, and
        platelet count
    Gross blood in stool on screening examination
    History of alcoholism or drug abuse

* The total volume of stones that can be treated has not been defined. Presumably, the smaller the volume, the better the results.

bladder, and a standard roentgenogram of the right upper quadrant to determine if the gallstones were calcified. In certain patients, CT scans of the gallbladder were performed. In women at risk for being pregnant, a beta-human chorionic gonadotropin was measured.

To be included in the study, the patient had to be considered a candidate for exploratory celiotomy and cholecystectomy should that prove to be necessary. The patient also had to be able to understand and comply with the study protocol, as well as being willing to give detailed informed consent. The criteria concerning the size of the stones and the ability of the gallbladder to concentrate contrast were strictly observed, as they have a bearing on the results. Sackmann and associates demonstrated that disruption of a solitary stone is easier than disruption of multiple stones, with 45% of patients with a small solitary stone being fragment-free 2 months after ESL combined with oral bile salt therapy.[11] Presumably, a functioning gallbladder is needed to extrude the stone fragments resulting from ESL.

The FDA's exclusion criteria were also observed. In particular, although preliminary evidence suggests that ESL can disrupt calcified stones, these fragments are not as responsive to the ursodeoxycholic acid therapy used in our protocol as are cholesterol fragments. Therefore, most patients with calcified stones seen on plain roentgenogram of the abdomen were excluded; those whose stones had only a thin eggshell rim or a small nidus of calcium were acceptable candidates.

Patient Population

In the BUMC experience, 579 patients were screened and 60 have been treated (10.4%). The most common cause of exclusion was lack of interest, defined as failure to complete the evaluation when not excluded by a deviation from the criteria (Table 2). The "other" category includes drug allergy, abnormalities of the screening test, pregnancy, drug or alcohol abuse, or bleeding disorders. These data correspond closely with those published in Germany, where 2,010 patients were screened, 565 (28%) were found to be appropriate candidates, and 175 (8.7%) were treated by ESL. As further experience is gained, patient selection can be expected to become more liberal.

Treatment

The BUMC protocol combines ESL and chemolysis with a bile salt supplement, ursodeoxycholic acid (Actigall; Ciba-Geigy). This naturally occurring bile acid decreases cholesterol secretion into bile, alters the cholesterol:phospholipid ratio of lipid vesicles secreted into the bile, and decreases

Table 2
Causes of Exclusion from ESL (N = 519)

	No. (%)
Lack of interest by patient	163 (31.4)
Inappropriate stone characteristics	
Too many stones	93 (17.9)
Inappropriate size	29 (5.4)
Presence of calcium	48 (9.2)
Patient not surgical candidate	38 (7.3)
Age outside limits	30 (5.8)
Nonopacification of gallbladder	26 (5.0)
Recent regional inflammatory change	8 (1.6)
Other	84 (16.2)

the absorption of dietary and biliary cholesterol.[12] Ursodiol also increases bile flow. The end result is a decreased biliary cholesterol saturation and increased flow through the system, causing a net absorption of cholesterol from stone fragments. Patients begin taking ursodeoxycholic acid in a dose of 10 mg/kg at least 7 days prior to ESL.

The Medstone 1050 machine used by BUMC is a flat, dry table without a water bath and has both ultrasound and x-ray localization capability, making it a truly dual-purpose machine for both gallstones and kidney stones. The shock wave generator is located beneath the table, and the patients are treated prone for cholelithiasis.

Initially, patients were admitted the night before ESL for final evaluation and sonographic evaluation to confirm that stones were still present. The following day, the patient was taken to the lithotripsy suite. The first 30 patients were treated under general endotracheal anesthesia. More recently, we have been admitting patients the day of the procedure and using intravenous analgesics without general anesthesia.

The patient's abdomen is shaved in order that maximum coupling can be achieved. The skin is bathed in mineral oil, as is the shield over the port in the table. It is important that no air be present in the shock wave path. Coupling is also accomplished between the table and the covering of the lens of the ellipsoid container from which the shock wave is generated.

Once the stone has been localized by ultrasonography, a light pen is used to identify the location of the stone for the computer, which directs positioning of the patient at the apex of the shock wave. If more than one stone is present, shock waves are distributed to each stone up to a maximum total of 2,000 shocks. Each time a different stone is treated, the patient is moved so that that stone is placed at the apex of the shock wave. Treatment lasts 45 to 90 minutes, depending on the number of stones and the number of relocalizations required. The patient is then placed back on a carrier and sent to the recovery room.

Patients can be discharged on the same day according to the approved FDA protocol. On the day after ESL, blood tests and sonography are repeated. All patients continue to receive ursodeoxycholic acid for as long as 3 months after they appear to have become stone-free to assist in the dissolution of fragments that might not pass spontaneously.

Results (see also Editors' Note, p. 101)

At BUMC, more than 60 patients have been treated during the past 8 months. With a follow-up averaging 4 months, more than 80% of the patients with solitary stones less than 2 cm are stone-free. Approximately 30% of patients had multiple stones, and 30% had two or three stones, and of these, approximately 15% are stone-free.

Gross, silent hematuria occurred in approximately 10% of patients. Some of the women who reported hematuria were menstruating, so the source of bleeding was not always clear. However, hematuria secondary to renal exposure to shock waves is known to occur.[13]

Approximately one-third of patients have mild, moderate, or occasionally, severe biliary colic, but few patients have required pain medication for relief. Only one patient has suffered acute cholecystitis and pancreatitis. One year earlier, this patient had had a similar episode of acute cholecystitis and pancreatitis necessitating hospitalization.

The largest available series of biliary ESL is that of

Sackmann and associates.[11] Of their 175 patients, 83% had a single stone. Between 430 and 1,600 shock waves were delivered with a treatment time ranging from 13 minutes to almost 3 hours. As in our series, the first several patients were treated under general anesthesia, but subsequent patients were treated with either intravenous or epidural anesthesia. Both chenodeoxycholic acid and ursodeoxycholic acid at doses of 7.5 mg/kg were administered as a single dose at bedtime beginning approximately 12 days prior to treatment and continuing for 3 months after the complete disappearance of all fragments. Only nine patients received ESL twice. Approximately 35% of the patients developed biliary pain, with 6% having biliary colic during their hospital stay. A few patients continued to have biliary colic for as long as 18 months. Only two patients had signs of mild pancreatitis, 1 month and 6 months following treatment.

Sixty-three percent of the patients in this German series were stone-free within 4 to 8 months and 91% within 12 to 18 months. The best results were obtained in patients with radiolucent gallstones 15 mm in diameter or less; 92% of these patients were free of stones in 12 months. In similar cases, litholytic therapy with ursodeoxycholic acid and chenodeoxycholic acid without lithotripsy produced a stone-free rate of only 38%.[14] By actuarial analysis, it is predicted that 83% of the patients with solitary stones up to 2 cm in diameter will be stone-free within 1 year after lithotripsy. Likewise, 72% of patients with stones 2 to 3 cm in diameter and 63% of those with two or three stones were expected to be stone-free at 1 year. A possible explanation for the fact that patients with multiple stones do not do as well as those with single stones is that a cloud of fragments may be produced by ESL in which remaining large fragments or other stones can be hidden.[11]

Conclusion

Because the gallbladder of a patient who has had stones is diseased and may have decreased motility, recurrence of stones is likely. Moreover, small fragments may remain after

ESL, creating a nidus for the development of new stones. After gallstone dissolution with bile salts, gallstones recur in as many as 40% of patients.[15,16] It is possible that treatment with oral bile salts will be successful or that with repeat ESL, the patient will again become stone-free.

Treatment of common bile duct stones by lithotripsy will require endoscopic papillotomy and insertion of a nasobiliary catheter for injection of contrast medium to locate the stone. As in the case of kidney stone localization, biplane image-intensified fluoroscopy will be needed. It will be necessary to avoid injury to the head of the pancreas. Given these problems, the first line of therapy for common duct stones will continue to be basket extraction through a previously formed T-tube tract or endoscopic sphincterotomy and basket extraction from below. ESL will probably be recommended only for poor-risk patients with stones greater than 20 mm.

Early in the clinical development of renal ESL, patient acceptance criteria were restrictive, and many patients still had stones after treatment. With further experience and research, more patients have become candidates, success rates have improved, and the rate of ESL in relation to new percutaneous and transurethral techniques is becoming more clear. A similar sequence of events can confidently be expected with biliary ESL. Some of the possibilities are discussed in Chapter 8.

References

1. Tyor MP: *Gallstone Disease.* Washington, DC. National Digestive Disease Education and Information Clearing House, Department of Health and Human Services, 1982.
2. Simeone JP, Ferrucci JT Jr: New trends in gallbladder imaging. *JAMA* 1981; 246:380.
3. Schoenfield L: Gallstones and other biliary diseases. *Ciba Clin Symp* 1982; 34:4.
4. Langebuch C: Ein Fall von Extirpation der Gallenblase wegen chronischer Cholelithiasis. *Berl Klin Wochenschr* 1882; 19:725.
5. Bachrach WH, Hoffman AF: Ursodeoxycholic acid in the treatment of cholesterol cholelithiasis. *Dig Dis Sci* 1982; 27:737.
6. Schoenfield LJ, Lachin JM, et al: Chenodiol (chenodeoxycholic

acid) for dissolution of gallstones. The National Cooperative Gallstones Study: A controlled study of efficacy and safety. *Ann Intern Med* 1981; 95:257.

7. Chaussy C, Schmiedt E, Jocham D, et al: First clinical experience with extracorporeal-induced destruction of kidney stones by shock waves. *J Urol* 1982; 127:417.

8. Brendel W, Enders G: Shock waves for gallstones: Animal studies. *Lancet* 1983; 1:1054.

9. Sauerbruch T, Delius M, Paumgartner G, et al: Fragmentation of gallstones by extracorporeal shock waves. *N Engl J Med* 1986; 314:818.

10. Sackmann M, Weber W, Delius M: Extracorporeal shock wave lithotripsy of gallstones without general anesthesia: First clinical experience. *Ann Intern Med* 1987; 107:348.

11. Sackmann M, Delius M, Sauerbruch T: Shock-wave lithotripsy of gallbladder stones: The first 175 patients. *N Engl J Med* 1988; 318:393.

12. Fromm H, Malavolti M: Dissolving gallstones. *Adv Intern Med* 1988; 33:411.

13. Rubin JI, Arger PH, Pollack HM, et al: Kidney changes after extracorporeal shock wave lithotripsy: CT evaluation. *Radiology* 1987; 162:21.

14. Podda M, Enders G, Zuin M, et al: Combined administration of ursodeoxycholic and chenodeoxycholic acid: A more effective way to dissolve radiolucent gallstones (abstract). *Gastroenterology* 1983; 84:1274.

15. Ruppin DC, Dowling RH: Is recurrence inevitable after gallstone dissolution by bile acid treatment? *Lancet* 1982; 23:181.

16. Dowling RH, Gleesome D, Ruppin DC, et al: Gallstone recurrence and post-dissolution management. In: Paumgartner G (ed): *Enterohepatic Circulation of Bile Acids and Sterol Metabolism,* Falk Symposium 42. Lancaster: MTP Press, 1985, p 361.

7

Operation of Lithotriptors

Henry C. Alder

Introduction

Extracorporeal shock wave lithotripsy (ESL) has rapidly become a routine alternative to kidney stone surgery, and recent experience with the treatment of ureteral stones with ESL suggests that this method can also substitute for some transureteral procedures (see Chapter 2). Therefore, it is not surprising that during the years from 1985 through 1988, the number of ESL facilities increased from six investigation sites to more than 200 operating facilities (Fig. 1). The number of facilities may easily double over the next 4 years, given ESL's potential new application for gallstones.

Lithotriptors are expensive. The current purchase price and installation costs often exceed $1.5 million, and incremental operating costs exceed $500,000 per year. Nevertheless, acquisition and operating costs have not been a significant barrier to the diffusion of this technology, as hospitals and physician groups have been creative in financing lithotriptors. The result has been a number of unique ventures and partnerships evidenced by the variety of operating configurations and ownerships of the lithotriptors in use today.

81

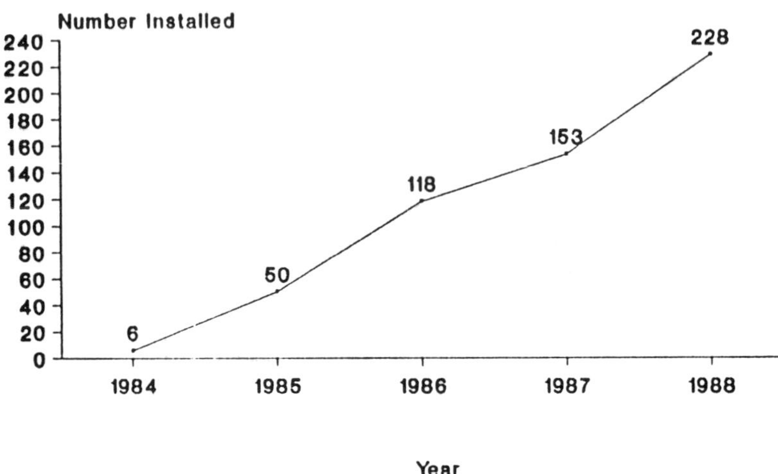

Figure 1: *Lithotriptor diffusion by year in the United States.*

This chapter will address the operating issues associated with lithotriptors so that providers—physicians and hospitals—can decide best how to implement this capability within their communities. There are several important factors, particularly ownership, patient volume projections, investment and operating costs, coverage and reimbursement, and facility utilization and competition for the treatment of stone patients. Each will be discussed.

Ownership

A lithotriptor survey conducted by the American Hospital Association (AHA) in 1987 showed that the predominant form of ownership for a lithotripsy facility was a joint venture or partnership (Table 1). In most cases, a hospital was the general partner, and other hospitals or physicians were limited partners. In addition, many free-standing and mobile lithotriptor facilities had been established by entrepreneurs or third parties. In these cases, the independent third party was the general partner, and limited partnerships were acquired by either hospitals or physicians.

Table 1

Lithotriptor Ownership*

Type	*Percent*
Joint venture	41.7
Hospital	22.9
Hospital chain	10.4
Physician group	8.3
Corporation	6.2
Foundation	6.2
Other	4.2

*Adapted from Alder HC, Murray ML: Operating Characteristics of U.S. Lithotriptor Facilities, AHA Hospital Technology Series Special Report, Chicago, American Hospital Association, 1987.

The structure of the ownership arrangement obviously differed from one operation to another. Strategically, hospitals developed partnerships with their urologists and other medical staff in order to avoid medical staff erosion and to increase physician loyalty. Similarly, hospitals cooperated with other hospitals (perhaps serving a market other than their own), recognizing that cooperation may be more profitable than attempting to compete for lithotripsy services.

Market pressures also encouraged the formation of partnerships. For instance, many hospitals are required to file certificate of need (CON) applications with state or regional health planners before initiating or reconfiguring a clinical service. The health regulatory agencies approve applications that demonstrate community need and curtail health care costs. Partnerships that share a new technology are approved more readily than are individual facility applications.

Patient Volume Projections

Projecting patient volume is important to assess the demand and average utilization of a shock wave lithotripsy facility. Patient volume can differ significantly from one region of the country to another. If the volume of patients who are candidates for lithotripsy is insufficient to recover the costs of the service at one site, perhaps alternatives to providing ESL at a single facility should be considered.

According to epidemiologists, the prevalence of kidney stone disease is approximately 2% to 3% of the adult population in Western industrialized nations and that of gallstones is approximately 10%. These data predict that about 2.2 million Americans have kidney stone disease and 20 million Americans have gallstone disease. However, not all sufferers of kidney stones and gallstones are hospitalized, seek medical attention, or even realize that they are stone formers until symptoms appear. Statistics from the National Health Survey–National Center for Health Statistics (NCHS) for 1986 (Table 2) indicate that a very small number (only 3.9%) of gallstone patients are hospitalized each year, yet a majority of these patients (63.9%) undergo a stone removal procedure. The kidney stone population is inclined to be hospitalized more frequently (about 19.4% of those with stones), but only a little more than a third (37.8%) of these patients undergo a stone removal procedure.

Patient volume projections can be based on prevalence data, but this method may introduce some error. As noted, the prevalence of kidney and gallbladder stone disease includes the entire population of stone formers, including those persons who may not know they have stone disease, and a spirited debate may arise about including such

---

Table 2

Prevalence and Volume of Treatments for Cholelithiasis and Urolithiasis, United States 1986*

	Cholelithiasis	*Urolithiasis*
U.S. prevalence	20 million	2.2 million
No. of inpatient discharges for condition	786,000	426,000
As percent of prevalence	3.9	19.4
Inpatient stone procedures	502,000	161,000
As percent of discharges	63.9	37.8

*National Center for Health Statistics: Detailed Diagnosis and Procedures for Patients Discharged From Short-Stay Hospitals, United States, 1986. National Health Survey Series 13, No. 95, Washington, DC, 1987.

Table 3

National Patient Volume Projections for Extracorporeal
Shock Wave Lithotripsy

	Cholelithiasis	*Urolithiasis*
Total hospital inpatient discharges (1986; NCHS)	786,000	426,000
Stone procedures per discharge (1986; NCHS)	0.639	0.378
ESL eligibility factor	0.30	0.50
ESL procedure	150,600	80,500*
As percent of hospital discharges	19.2	18.9

*Outpatient ESL procedures performed at freestanding sites and mobile lithotriptors are not included in this projection. It is expected that outpatient lithotripsy procedures would increase this figure by at least 50% to more than 120,000 procedures per year.

patients in a model to forecast lithotripsy patient volume. Realistic volume projections are better estimated from inpatient discharge and procedure data. A model of patient volume projections can be constructed from current stone procedure experience, and Table 3 shows one method to determine demand given historical stone procedure data from a recognized data source (NCHS) and an estimated ESL substitution rate (ESL eligibility factor). As shown, the projected ESL inpatient volume is about 19% of hospital discharges for cholelithiasis as well as urolithiasis. Using 1986 hospital discharge data as representative, one can assume that each year, 80,500 urolithiasis inpatients and 150,600 cholelithiasis inpatients could be eligible for ESL.

This model, like all models for projecting patient volume, makes a number of assumptions to simplify calculations. These assumptions include: (1) all lithotripsy treatment in the hospital only (no outpatient or free-standing treatments), (2) lithotriptors are distributed uniformly throughout United States based on population and need, and (3) all physicians and patients have access to ESL. The effects of these assumptions must be factored into any analysis.

Investment and Operating Costs

The investment and operating costs of a lithotriptor are significant. Indeed, for many hospitals and physicians, they may be a barrier to providing ESL services. To operate a lithotriptor facility successfully, the costs should be identified, and a plan should be developed to obtain payback as soon as possible.

Numerous firms offer a variety of lithotriptor configurations and prices, although only three companies with Food and Drug Administration (FDA) lithotriptors—Dornier Medical Systems (Atlanta, GA), Medstone (Costa Mesa, CA), and Siemens (Iselin, NJ)—are permitted to sell their devices at the time of this writing. The prices of their lithotriptors are $1.5 million, $1.4 million, and $1.4 million, respectively. Other market entrants have investigational device exemptions (IDEs) to perform gallstone and kidney stone clinical trials. A brief description with prices of these second- and third-generation lithotriptors is provided in Table 4. As can be seen, the prices of later-generation devices are expected to be $1 million or less. Surely these devices will attract those hospitals and physicians whose patient volume projections would not allow them to realize an appropriate return on the more expensive lithotriptors.

Lithotriptor operating costs encompass a variety of direct and indirect costs, including professional and support staff salaries, insurance, telephone, maintenance contracts, space, and medical supplies (such as electrodes). Actual operating costs differ significantly from one facility to another, depending on the resources required to support the lithotriptor. On average, the direct costs for a lithotriptor are approximately $500,000 per year.

Hospitals and physician groups that operated lithotriptor facilities in 1986 reported in a 1987 AHA lithotriptor survey that their average cost per procedure was $2,900. Assuming they were able to obtain full payment for their costs, these facilities reported that they would be required to treat 650 patients per year to break even.

Table 4
Lithotriptor Status and Prices*

Manufacturer	Model	FDA Status	Approximate Price ($Millions)
Diasonics	Therasonic	IDE Kidney	?
Direx (Israel)	Tripter X 1	IDE Kidney	0.30
Dornier Medical Systems	HM-3	PMA Kidney IDE Common duct	1.70
	HM-4	PMA Kidney	1.50
	MFL 5000	IDE Kidney	
	MPL 9000	IDE Gallbladder	1.0
EDAP	Lithedap LT.01.	IDE Kidney IDE Gallbladder	0.75
Medstone	1050ST	PMA Kidney IDE Gallbladder	1.40
Nitech (Denmark)	?	?	?
Northgate Research	SD-3	IDE Kidney IDE Gallbladder	0.40
Siemens	Lithostar	PMA Kidney IDE Common duct	1.40
Technomed	Sonolith 2000	IDE Kidney	0.95
	Sonolith 3000	IDE Kidney IDE Common Duct IDE Gallbladder	?
Wolf	Piezolith 2200	IDE Kidney IDE Gallbladder	0.95
Yashihoda (Japan)	SZ-1	?	1.40

*Status and prices as of December, 1988.

Coverage and Reimbursement

Coverage and reimbursement are a serious concern for providers in the present era of shrinking payments. One of the concerns associated with a lithotripsy service is to determine the payment providers may recover from third-party payers.

Hospitals and free-standing lithotriptor facilities that responded to the 1987 AHA lithotriptor survey indicated that the predominant payers for lithotripsy are commercial carriers (43%), Blue Cross/Blue Shield plans (25%), and Medicare (19%). The commercial carriers and Blue Cross/

Blue Shield plans reimburse for inpatient and outpatient lithotripsy based on the facility's charges less a discount or some negotiated rate. Medicare reimburses inpatient lithotripsy based on DRGs (except in those states with waivers) but does not reimburse for outpatient ESL.

Coverage and reimbursement is unavailable from most carriers during lithotriptor clinical trials. As a result, payment responsibility must be determined prior to treatment. The payment policy for investigation sites varies. Several IDE sites have required patients to assume full responsibility for payment. These patients must negotiate with their own health insurance carrier to receive reimbursement for their hospitalization and treatment. Other investigation sites have assumed the role of patient advocate and will negotiate directly with a health insurance carrier to ascertain coverage and recover reimbursement. Because ESL is recognized as a potential cost-saving technology, some investigation sites have obtained payment from more than 70% of their major payers to cover 90% of the hospital's charges.

Medicare coverage and payment is governed by the Health Care Financing Administration (HCFA). Generally, HCFA considers coverage policy on new technology only after the technology has been approved by the FDA and has begun to be diffused.

The Blue Cross/Blue Shield plans provide coverage after clinical trials have been accepted and fully approved by the FDA. However, individual plans make independent coverage determinations. Giving overwhelmingly positive clinical information about the efficacy of a new technology may encourage some plans to make coverage determination decisions prior to FDA approval.

Facility Utilization and Competition for the Treatment of Stone Patients

A number of significant marketplace dynamics have begun to impact decisions to provide lithotripsy services. As a result of the rapid diffusion of this technology for kidney stones, a saturation effect has begun to appear. The slowly increasing pool of kidney stone patients eligible for

Table 5
Average Monthly Lithotriptor Procedures by Year of Installation*

	1984 Adopter	*1985 Adopter*	*1986 Adopter*	*Percent of Change in Procedure Volume (1986 compared to 1984)*
First year of operation	148	77	57	39
October 1986	109	77	60	55
Percent change	−26	0	+5	

*From: Alder HC, Murray ML: Operating Characteristics of U.S. Lithotriptor Facilities, AHA Hospital Technology Series Special Report, Chicago, American Hospital Association, 1987.

treatment is being spread among an ever-larger pool of providers. This phenomenon was evident in the 1987 AHA lithotriptor survey, which showed that later lithotriptor acquirers had patient populations as small as 39% of those of their counterparts who acquired lithotriptors 2 years earlier. Early acquirers also experienced a decline in patient numbers of as much as 26% after 2 years of operation (Table 5).

While increasing diffusion decreased utilization, another phenomenon also impacted initial utilization: pent-up demand. Urologists predicted that lithotriptor utilization would decrease within 2 or 3 years because the early adopters would deplete those kidney stone patients who had postponed elective stone surgery 1 or 2 years or more anticipating the availability of a kidney stone lithotriptor. Because kidney stones often do not recur for 5 to 10 years, the only patients who would remain would be those with difficult stones that cannot be treated by ESL, those patients who are at risk for any type of procedure requiring anesthesia (although currently available anesthesia-free lithotriptors may be used for these patients), and those patients in whom kidney stones recur frequently. New patients would emerge each year as eligible lithotripsy patients as the population slowly ages.

This scenario is expected to be replayed in the treatment of gallstones. Early biliary lithotripsy providers will treat large numbers of eligible gallstone patients, at least initially. However, as more lithotriptor facilities come online, the supply of patients to be treated will be distributed among a greater number of facilities. Late biliary lithotriptor adopters will be at a disadvantage because they have not had the opportunity to build experience or promote their uniqueness to their service area. They will be at an additional disadvantage if the late adopters purchase lithotriptor technology at the same price as the early adopters. They will be able to compete effectively for stone patients only by either pooling their resources with other providers in a joint venture or partnership or by acquiring a low-priced, later-generation machine.

8

Status and Future Role of Biliary Lithotripsy

LeRoy H. Stahlgren

Introduction

Will the success of lithotripsy in the treatment of renal stones be translated into equally good results with gallstones?

Despite the striking similarities in rates of stone fragmentation and the similar lack of significant tissue damage in response to extracorporeal shock wave lithotripsy (ESL), important dissimilarities exist between these organ systems. For example, the biliary tract is anatomically more complex. The gallbladder acts as a stone-containing reservoir or appendage that resides outside the main stream of bile flow. Moreover, bile flow is modest in quantity and traverses a low-pressure conduit with limited contractility. For these reasons, gallstone fragments may not clear as readily as those of renal stones and may be more difficult to retrieve endoscopically should that be required. Adjunctive litholytic therapy may reduce but will not eliminate such concerns. An additional dissimilarity is the expendability of the diseased gallbladder, a characteristic obviously not shared by

91

the kidneys. Cholecystectomy does not compromise the digestive process, nor does it pose a significant health threat.

In the patients' view, the feature common to the lithotriptor treatment of both types of stones and which drives its use is the avoidance of surgery and postoperative disability. But will biliary lithotripsy replace cholecystectomy? To compare lithotripsy with surgery properly requires detailed examination of risk, efficacy, and cost.

Risk

To date, there have been no deaths and only rare complications attributed to lithotripsy. The incidence of stone fragment complications is only 1% to 2% and that of biliary pain is approximately 30%.[1] Adjunctive chemolytic therapy (ursodeoxycholic acid 8 to 10 mg/kg daily) uncommonly causes consequential diarrhea or changes in liver function studies.[2]

Mortality rates for the half-million cholecystectomies performed annually in the United States range from 0.08% to 4.2%.[3] The higher rates may be irrelevant to this discussion, as those series included high-risk older patients suffering from stone complications and coincident medical disorders; objectivity requires that only like cases be compared, and no such poor-risk patients currently undergo lithotripsy. When the subset of patients identified in the lithotriptor protocol is considered, operative death occurs in only one in 500 to one in 1,000 elective cholecystectomies, and many surgeons can point to a zero mortality rate after thousands of such procedures. Operative mortality thus should not, in itself, figure as a major deterrent to elective cholecystectomy.

Surgical complications, including biliary (10.4%) and nonbiliary (5.9%) problems, do not usually seriously compromise the patient.[4,5] However, all surgery patients experience stress, discomfort, and disability. In that regard, lithotripsy offers advantages over surgery for the specific subset of patients who are part of existing lithotriptor protocols. Such quality of life issues will be discussed under *Cost.*

Efficacy

Cholecystectomy is nearly 100% effective in patients who would also be candidates for ESL. Retained stones and common duct explorations are so rare in such cases as to be discounted. Some authors have focused attention on the 20% to 30% incidence of postcholecystectomy symptoms, but when examined carefully, such symptoms can usually be attributed to the persistence of preexisting disorders. To the extent that patients with nonbiliary complaints such as heartburn, bloating, indigestion, and dyspepsia are subjected to cholecystectomy or, for that matter, to lithotripsy, there will be patients who do not become asymptomatic. Poor case selection is responsible for such failures, not the treatment itself.

At least three dimensions of success must be surveyed when evaluating the results of lithotripsy: stone fragmentation, stone clearance, and stone recurrence.

Fragmentation

To date, nearly 100% of protocol-selected stones have disintegrated with ESL.[1] Such success may well lead to broadening of the criteria for acceptable stone characteristics as to size, number, and degree of calcification.

Clearance

Stone clearance rates are similar to those with renal lithotripsy, i.e., more than 90% clear with adjunctive chemolytic therapy.[1] Despite such results, treatment failure rates exceed those of elective cholecystectomy. Operation is curative in that the stones and the organ in which they are formed are eliminated permanently.

Recurrence

Recognizing that long-term follow-up data are insufficient to predict recurrence after lithotripsy, one may look for guidance to the results after dissolution therapy. Recurrence after such treatment approaches 50% in 5 years.[2] Existing data do not permit one to predict whether larger and fewer stones recur less frequently than numerous small stones. However, knowledge of stone pathophysiology supports the expectation that stones will re-form in at least some patients because the circumstances persist that first led to stone formation.

Further progress in understanding gallstone pathophysiology may lead to new methods of stone prevention. Such developments may be required before recurrence after ESL is ultimately controlled. Currently, the only clinically available method of inhibition of stone formation is bile salt therapy, and long-term litholytic therapy is problematic because of cost. New stones may, of course, be treated by repeat lithotripsy.

Cost

During the investigational phase of ESL, protocol-directed laboratory and imaging tests artificially inflate costs. For comparison of expenditures, we will assume Food and Drug Administration approval of lithotripsy and adjunctive litholytic therapy. Cost comparisons at a large private teaching hospital are tabulated in Table 1.

The direct costs of ESL are marginally higher than those of operation. More difficult to calculate are the quality-of-life issues associated with operation and postoperative disability that are not a concern with ESL. The cost of 1 month's disability can be readily calculated for an individual but is much more difficult to assess when large numbers are involved, as the mix of occupations represented by the half-million patients undergoing operations may or may not reflect societal norms. To take one example, the estimated cost of replacing a housewife's services may reach or exceed $48,000 annually. Therefore, 1 month's disability should add an additional $4,000 to the housewife's surgical bill. Whatever the figure, society pays considerably for lost productivity whether in the home or in the work force.

Considering that the mortality rate for elective cholecystectomy ranges from 0.1% to 0.5%, and estimating that

Table 1
Comparison of Costs ($) of Treatment Modalities

	Lithotripsy	*Surgery*	*Litholytic*
Pretreatment imaging			
Ultrasound	145	145	145
X-ray	60	—	60
OCG	100	—	100
Total	305	145	305
Post-treatment			
Ultrasound	290	—	720*
Hospitalization	4000	4440	—
Professional	2000	2000	330 (four visits)
Ursodiol	545		1090
Total	7140	6585	2445
Lost productivity (days)	1–2	30[+]	Office visits only
Mortality rate (%)	0	0.1–0.5	0
Complication rate (%)	2	10–16	0
Recurrence rate (%)	?	0–1	50 (at 5 years)

*Scans at 1, 3, 6, 9, and 12 months.
[+] Estimated cost for a typical patient: $4000 (see text).

approximately 400,000 such nonemergency operations are performed annually in the United States, between 400 and 2,000 patients unexpectedly die postoperatively each year. The years of lost life expectancy, if calculated to be 28 years per death, may amount to 60,000 years annually (average age at operation = 50; estimated life expectancy at 50 years of age is 28 years).[6]

The principal advantage of operation is its finality. Patients will not be troubled further with gallbladder disease. Treatment is a one-time affair requiring no further follow-up once recovery has occurred. Such may not be the case after lithotripsy. Repeated ESL or cholecystectomy may become necessary if stones recur. That risk can be neither predicted nor assessed at this time. In choosing between lithotripsy and operation in a carefully selected subset of patients, one must balance the benefits of the minimal impact on the patient's general health and productivity of the former against the definitive nature of the latter. For the present, patients are volunteering for ESL in the clinical trials and are accepting lithotripsy as an alternative to surgery with knowledge of the uncertainties described above. It is not expected that lithotripsy will replace operation for patients with acute cholecystitis, obstructive jaundice, or nonfunctioning gallbladder. Lithotripsy may become marginally useful in treatment of large stone volumes and calcified stones. As such cases represent the majority of the half-million patients operated on each year, lithotripsy may be applicable to only 20% to 30%. Nonetheless, 20% of a half-million cases represents a considerable population. (See Figure 1 for a treatment algorithm.)

Conclusion

It is clear that treatment of gallstones is no longer unidimensional and is no longer exclusively the province of the surgeon. Endoscopists, interventional radiologists, and researchers have entered the field, and their collective efforts promise to enlarge considerably the available therapeutic options.

In the post-IDE period, ESL will probably be extended

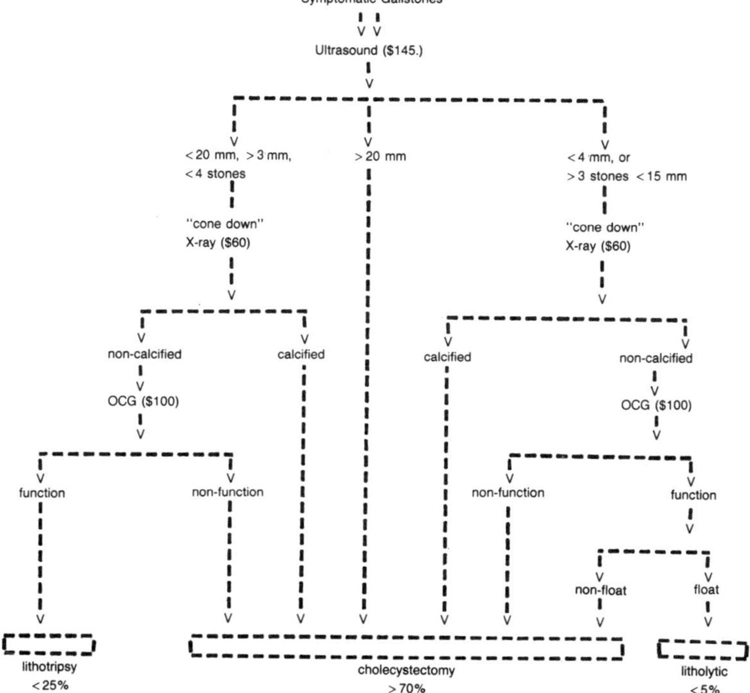

Figure 1: *Algorithm for management of symptomatic gallstones.*

to poor-risk and older patients. Treatment of selected
asymptomatic patients may also be considered. With the
risk of complications developing in patients with certain
types of silent stones, "preventive" treatment may be considered, particularly in older patients. Surgeons will remain
the major, but not the only, players in a field which they
previously dominated. Nevertheless, surgical treatment,
which has been tested for more than 100 years, will prevail
as the gold standard against which all new modalities are
measured.

APPENDIX

Food and Drug Administration (FDA) Procedures for Considering Lithotripsy Proposals, Illustrated by the History of Medstone's Application

October 1987

Application filed for Investigational Device Exemption (IDE) and Investigational New Drug Exemption (IND). The FDA is required to respond within 30 days to such applications with one of three options: approval, rejection, or recommendation. In this instance, the FDA requested additional safety data based on animal trials. Such data were obtained and submitted.

January 1988

The FDA approved the IDE and IND, the number of investigational sites (7), and the number of cases (200). Clinical trials began on January 27. The time elapsed from submission to approval, including additional animal trials, thus was approximately 4 months. The IDE process requires documentation of safety, mechanical integrity, management expertise, and appropriateness of protocol.

Spring 1989 (estimate)

Application for premarket approval (PMA). Upon Medstone's expected submission of data from 200 cases, the FDA will conduct an initial review within 45 days. The FDA's options are to rule the application nonfileable (deficient and not worthy of exhaustive review) or fileable. If the application is accepted for filing, the FDA conducts an in-depth internal review. Part of that process includes a convened public forum to which are invited outside experts, company representatives, and other interested individuals. The FDA's options then include full approval, rejection, or approval with conditions.

References

1. Sackmann M, Delius M, Sauerbruch T, et al: Shock-wave lithotripsy of gallbladder stones: The first 175 patients. *N Engl J Med* 1988; 318:393.
2. Fromm H: Gallstone dissolution and therapy. *Gastroenterology* 1986; 91:1560.
3. McSherry CK, Glenn F: The incidence and causes of death following surgery for non-malignant biliary tract disease. *Ann Surg* 1980; 191:271.
4. Sandler RS, Maule WF, Baltus ME: Factors associated with postoperative complications in diabetics after biliary tract surgery. *Gastroenterology* 1986; 91:157.
5. DenBesten L, Berie G: The current status of biliary tract surgery: An international study of 1072 consecutive patients. *World J Surg* 1986; 10:116.
6. US Department of Health and Human Services: Vital Statistics of the US, 1985; Life Tables, vol 11, section 6. Washington, DC: USDHHS, 1988.

Editors' Note: Results in 266 Patients Treated with Medstone Biliary Lithotriptor 1050

The Medstone International FDA-approved IDE trial started in January 1988 at Baylor University Medical Center, Dallas, Texas. During 1988, the other nine fixed sites, listed below, were installed and began treating patients:

- University of Nebraska, Omaha, Nebraska
- Tulane University, New Orleans, Louisiana
- Abbott-Northwestern Hospital, Minneapolis, Minnesota
- Baptist Memorial Hospital, Memphis, Tennessee
- Cabrini Medical Center, New York, New York
- St. Joseph's Hospital, Denver, Colorado
- University of Pittsburgh, Pittsburgh, Pennsylvania
- Mount Carmel Hospital, Columbus, Ohio
- University of Kansas, Kansas City, Kansas

The mobile sites (being organized now) are:

- Baptist Medical Centers of Birmingham, Alabama, and surrounding hospitals
- Network of Southern Californian Hospitals

Patient Data

In the 266 patients, the age range was 19 to 77 years with the average being approximately 45 years. One-third were men; 94% were white. Patient weight ranged from 90 to 350 pounds, with the average being 172 pounds.

Stone Data

Approximately half the patients had solitary gallstones, 30% had two or three stones, and 20% had more than three stones. Sixty percent of the stones were 1 to 2 cm. 20% were smaller than 1 cm, and 20% were greater than 2 cm. Ninety-five percent of the patients did not show stone calcification.

Results and Complications

The fragmentation rate was 95%. All of the patients had biliary colic prior to treatment, and after treatment approximately half the patients had biliary colic. Skin ecchymosis was noted in about one-quarter of the patients and resolved within 3 to 5 days. In some patients, there was mild elevation of liver and pancreatic enzymes, which, again, resolved within the first 3 days in almost all of the cases. One patient had ERCP with removal of fragments from the distal common duct, and two patients underwent cholecystectomy because of partial blockage of the cystic duct secondary to stone fragments. No other significant side effects were noted. No patients died.

Follow-Up

For patients with solitary stones less than 2 cm in size, the observed cumulative stone-free rate at 6 months was 85%. This compares favorably with the Munich experience in 175 patients treated with a Dornier lithotriptor where patients with solitary stones less than 2 cm in size were stone-free in 78% 4 to 8 months after ESL.[1]

Reference

1. Sackmann M, Delius M, Sauerbruch T, et al: Shockwave lithotripsy of gallbladder stones: The first 175 patients. *N Engl J Med* 1988; 318:393.

Index